FUNCTIONAL FITNESS™

The Ultimate Fitness Program for Life on The Run

• • • • • • • • • • • •

Larkin Barnett

FAP BOOKS
FLORIDA ACADEMIC PRESS, INC.
Gainesville and London

Thanks to:

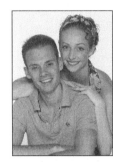

Callie Manning and Didier Bramaz, Soloists with Miami City Ballet

ON THE COVER:
Callie Manning

Contributors:
Exercise Photography thanks to Ray Graham © 2005

Dance Photography thanks to Steven Caras © 2005,
Director of Development, Miami City Ballet

Book design by Kristen Bergman Morales

Illustrations by Caren Hackman, carenhackman.com

Special thanks to the editors MG Owens, Allie Hanley, Jennifer Marcello, Mario Burbano, Paul Medas, Griffin Barnett, Blake Barnett, as well as Howard Gitten, Bruce Taylor, Roz Usheroff, Tricia Cristafulli, Diane Crovo, Glorianna Peale, Claude Rozinsky and Elena Fasulo.

FUNCTIONAL FITNESS™

The Ultimate Fitness Program for Life on The Run

Principles of Movement Come Alive Through Imagery and
Experiential Anatomy for Pilates, Sports, Dance, Gym Workouts, and Daily Life

Larkin Barnett

Published in the United States of America by Florida Academic Press,
Gainesville, FL, March 2006

Library of Congress Control Number: 200692124

Cover art with permission by Ray Graham
Cover prepared by Kristen Bergman Morales

The Life Extension System, Athletickinetic Recipe, The Amazing Sock Ball,
Three-Dimensional Breathing, and The Foundation Exercise are trademarks
or registered trademarks of Larkinetics Inc.

For more information visit: www.larkinetics.com
or E-mail: info@larkinetics.com

For Eija Celli, my dance professor

PART ONE

Preface

Being a motivational speaker to many corporations, the mind coach of professional athletes, and a relationship trainer, it is of utmost importance to be clear and precise. I concentrate on how the brain processes. If the belief system is not beneficial for the individual, I show methods for eliciting change to beliefs that are. When things have worked well for so long, people tend to think that it always will. They don't take new information and situations into account.

The exciting news is that Larkin Barnett has written a book that does just that. She has created The Life Extension System, which takes new information and combines it with current fitness methods. She has clarified the basic truths of the principles of movement derived from various experts in the field of movement and dance. She then took quantum leaps to combine the mental, emotional, spiritual, and physical components of movement to benefit even the newcomer to exercise.

It is important to know some of the history of these movement innovators. Before coming to America in 1926, Joseph Pilates worked with European pioneers of movement, although he was closest to Rudolf Laban.

While Pilates felt that within each of us resides an "inner athlete," Laban believed that deep down everyone is a dancer. Pilates shared Laban's ideas with his body conditioning method and offered it to prominent dance circles. Pilates training impressed George Balanchine, particularly in regard to injured dancers. Laban was a movement theorist who pondered the why and how of the craft of dance. Among many of his contributions is a systematic analysis of the body moving in space. He felt that true dance forms spring from the body's sense of time and space. This book sets the groundwork for Laban's work to be a part of every Pilates practitioner's literacy.

In Pilates it is equally important to strengthen muscle groups while thinking in terms of the entire body as a unit moving through space. This produces maximum functioning—a body that moves with ease and efficiency. Larkin's recipe and simple introduction to spatial concepts requires intention and awareness on the part of the Pilates participant. Then the individual is no longer just practicing the physical components of the exercise, but they can feel the more expressive aspects of a dancer in motion.

Larkin's mentor Eija Celli studied with many of the original students of Laban, as well as Martha Graham and Merce Cunningham, some of the pioneers of modern dance. These proprietary exercises created in the 1970s are a result of Larkin's foundation in her early dance training. Eija Celli is a dance historian who has continued the expansion of Laban's work through the scientific aspects of dance, including dynamic alignment. At the core of Eija Celli's teaching is the belief that when a dancer, fitness participant, or even someone doing rehabilitation moves their body with a conscious use of the space around them it immediately involves intention and concentration, resulting in the beauty of their very essence or spirit expressing itself.

Now there is an outstanding book that highlights the theories of both Pilates and Laban. Larkin's user-friendly exercises embody the spatial elements from Laban's work and combine it in a fun, exciting way with Pilates through the use of creative visualization. Instead of sheer muscular strength the exercises gently guide us to more efficient, sequential movements. We can all move with the efficiency of an athlete, grace of a dancer, and the fluidity and power of an animal.

Larkin's insightful, scientific-based visual imagery provides precise ways of working with the body. She created The Life Extension System for balance, vitality, and longevity. It gives us a resource to live in our body with supple muscles and emotional calmness. Her intimate knowledge of the body is crucial for the athlete and dancer. This book is a tremendous resource of both inspiration and information.

Larkin's imagery is extraordinary. She uses it to reinforce and integrate concepts for rehabilitation, preventative health, dancers, athletes, and for the layperson. This Pilates-based lifestyle is a handbook for our needs while we go about our busy lives. The American Heart Association recommends 30 minutes of moderate exercise, most days each week. Research shows that you are better off accumulating about 30 minutes of physical activity each day—10 minutes here, 5 minutes there—without losing any of the health benefits. These mini workouts that can be done throughout the course of the day are the key to fitness within our busy lifestyles.

The use of imagery in all areas of movement has grown in large part due to dancers and athletes' success with visualization. It is a common practice for an athlete to close their eyes and visualize the actions of their event, as well as standing on the podium winning their medal. This book is a powerful tool for movement specialists to use in their work. The humor and clarity in which the ideas are conveyed makes it easily understandable even without a scientific background. It enriches whatever endeavors we are pursuing in the movement arena. Imaging can alter the physiology and neuromuscular behavior of the body that results in correcting inappropriate habitual movement patterns.

Larkin takes imagery and combines aspects of anatomy, physiology, and biomechanics and its application to actual fitness exercises. She moves us through the imaging while we physically do exercises that are combining disciplines from massage, reflexology, breathing techniques, and methods from the martial arts. There has been nothing up to this time that is as clear, precise, and comprehensive as this book. I applaud Larkin Barnett for giving birth to this wonder, something for all of us to make use of as a valuable resource.

Dr. Madeleine Singer, PhD.

Introduction

BUSY BANK LINE BLUES

Recently, I walked into the bank, and there were twenty people waiting in line. There was only one teller, who was extremely stressed out. Merely glancing at the faces in the crowded line made her jaw clench tighter. The people were displaying predictable signs of frustration. One man was shifting his weight from one leg to the other, and his eyes furtively darted about. A mother with raised shoulders sighed while her child tugged at her skirt. Others kept nervously checking their watches or stood very still, with tightly crossed arms. The air was thick with impatience.

I was reminded of why I designed these exercises. It was for a situation like this. My mind-body visual imagery exercises could have turned these discontented expressions into smiles. I made a decision not to let this busy bank line get the best of me. I decided to go through a little routine—my own private workout.

Relaxing sensations ran up my spine to my neck. This allowed me to energize my body a bit more with **Three-Dimensional Breathing**. Then I aligned my **Pelvis as a Fish Bowl**, and toned up my abdominal muscles with **The Foundation Exercise**. I finished by balancing myself with **The Compass**. This routine helped

THREE-DIMENSIONAL BREATHING

See Page 74

PELVIS AS A FISH BOWL

See Page 56

THE FOUNDATION EXERCISE

See Page 83

THE COMPASS

See Page 52

PILATES

Combines the mind and body to access the deeper layers of postural muscles.

pass the time until I arrived at the teller—30 minutes later. Focusing on exercise instead of the wait had kept the slightest tension out of my body. I left the bank feeling relaxed and energized.

In our time-deprived society, it is a necessity to have a fitness program that can be done while on the run. Especially one that focuses on the principles of movement from the ancient disciplines of yoga and the martial arts—now essential for success in fitness, sports, and Pilates.

WHAT IS PILATES?

Joseph Pilates (1880-1967), the originator of the Pilates method of exercise, was a fitness trainer. Joseph devoted himself to a lifelong study of human physiology. His exercises create a balanced physique and help correct existing weaknesses in the body. In a world where health advice changes on a regular basis, Pilates remains reliable. Other fitness systems tend to concentrate on superficial muscles with the intention of building bulk. Pilates uses the mind as well as the body to help you achieve your goals. Pilates accesses the deeper layers of postural muscles. The end product of this *Functional Fitness* training is the strength, grace, and lean muscles of a dancer.

Joseph established his New York City studio in 1926, after moving from Europe. It attracted such innovative modern dancers as Martha Graham and ballet master George Balanchine.

Joseph Pilates' method was a combination of many disciplines. Joseph studied and practiced dance, yoga, and the martial arts. The method emphasizes the principles of movement present in all of these disciplines.

The fitness program in this book contains an easy presentation of the essential alignment, breathing, and centering principles. The exercises can be performed in conjunction with more organized events, such as sports, or with activities we do every day. With this easy-to-implement approach your fitness program can come first. The benefits include toned abdominal muscles, flexibility, coordination, and balance. You use visualization to develop longer, leaner muscles and have an overall gracefulness to your everyday movements.

MIND-BODY CONNECTION

All athletes incorporate the use of visualization into their training to enhance physical skills and attain goals. Joseph Pilates was a consummate athlete. He was an accomplished boxer, swimmer, gymnast, diver, and skier. Many of his exercises mimic the movements of sports. It was Joseph's dream that everyone discover his or her own "inner athlete." Every ex-

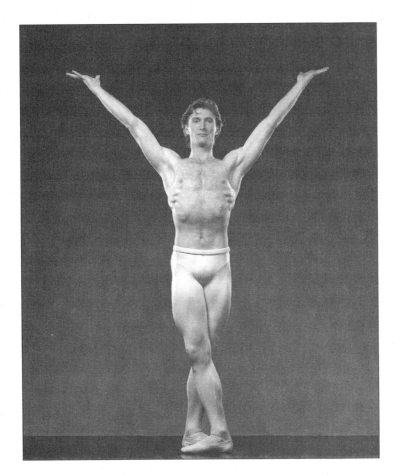

The end product of this Functional Fitness training is the strength, grace, and lean muscles of a dancer.

Mikhail Nikitine,
Miami City Ballet Soloist

Photograph:
© Steven Caras, 2005

ercise in this book will teach you how to use visualization to hasten the changes in your body or train for athletic success. Pilates requires the same level of control as sports. It takes a lot of control to place a tennis ball just inside the line, or to execute the perfect ski turn. Visualization helps you do the exercises carefully. You focus your effort, get more benefit from the movement, and progress quicker. This is the perfect conditioning program for any sport or a great way to get in shape.

The mind-body connection is what makes Pilates a unique form of fitness training. By controlling your mind you can change your body. Visual imagery is the pathway to understanding the fundamentals of Pilates. This program emphasizes practicing and breaking down the components behind the Pilates method. Refining the concepts and activating your mind-body connection throughout the day provides more understanding, safety, and results for the mat work.

Visual imagery makes it possible to integrate the building blocks of Pilates directly into your daily activities. The result is a deeper appreciation of the legacy of the Pilates method. Pilates continues to evolve. The Pilates-based work encompasses many variations. Most leaders in the field of Pilates, and even those who studied with Joseph Pilates in

THE PROGRAM

These exercises can be incorporated into your daily chores and office work — standing, sitting, lying down, or walking.

VISUALIZATION

By focusing your effort, you get more benefit from your movement and progress quicker.

15

the last years of his life continue to modify the method. They devised programs that make the work accessible to ordinary people and those recovering from injuries. This contemporary approach honors the original Pilates philosophy while taking into consideration advancements in scientific fitness training. This makes it necessary to have a thorough understanding of its original principles. Pilates principles adapt smoothly into everyday activities through the use of visualization exercises. You may decide to participate in Pilates in a studio, or while traveling. No two Pilates classes are the same. This program also allows you to become adept at integrating the key principles into any setting.

PRINCIPLES OF MOVEMENT FOR YOUR EVERYDAY ACTIVITIES

This is a program that encapsulates the essential principles of movement present in not only Pilates, but also in dance, yoga, and the martial arts. You can practice them anytime, anywhere, throughout your day—without machines. Integration of these exercises into your everyday activities reinforces important fitness concepts. Persistent practice of these principles during your normal day-to-day life prepares your mind and body for more success on the mat.

Joseph Pilates felt his mat exercises positively enhanced the participants' daily fitness. He said, "Our bodies are slumped, our shoulders are stooped, our eyes are hollow, our muscles are flabby and our vitality extremely lowered, if not vanished. This is but the natural result of not having uniformly developed all the muscles of our spine, trunk, arms, and legs in the course of pursuing our daily labors and office activities."

This is a program of easy-to-follow exercises to incorporate into your chores, errands, and office work. They can be practiced while standing, sitting, lying down, or walking. You will stop feeling robbed of energy by the end of a hectic day. You gain physical stamina and mental acuity. The principles of movement are clarified for you with this travel program of easy-to-implement mini-workouts. With this approach, Pilates is more than an exercise method: it is a way of life. Many with the desire but not the time to do Pilates can now take the first step.

You can ease into the practice of Pilates without taking a ton of time out of your day. The visual imagery provides a smooth transition to "jump start" you on a program of exercise. It is a fun way of adding exercises to your everyday experiences—watching television, at the park, or even while at your desk. This is an easy to follow, progressive fitness program. By paying attention to your posture, breathing, and abdominal muscles throughout the normal course of your day, you are facilitating results in your Desk Freedom or mat programs.

These exercises promote the mental practice of using a visual image to improve your motor skills. Mind-body visual imagery exercises play a key role in increasing efficiency of motion. The imagery exercises help you to activate and engage your muscles—not tense or grip them. This results in a healthier body and the potential for a more active life.

The average adult spends the day sitting in uncomfortable positions while commuting or working. The body's natural range of movement becomes restricted. It becomes vital to stretch and exercise in order to offset the effects of daily life. Visual imagery has the amazing potential to release physical and mental tension. By taking just a few minutes each day for these easy, empowering exercises—wherever you may be—you will be rewarded with a stronger and more agile body. These exercises increase your awareness of alignment and breathing while simultaneously building your muscle groups.

Visual imagery and fitness make a strong team. It will improve your memory, optimism, energy, self-esteem, sleep patterns, and relaxation. Imagery is a fun way to develop the power of your mind and body to dramatically improve your posture, flexibility, and balance, enhance your physical strength, mental focus, and emotional equilibrium for a better quality of life.

How to use the Book

The following guide boxes are located throughout the book.

VISUAL IMAGERY ▶
GUIDE

The Foundation for Understanding the Basic Movement Principles of Pilates, Dance, Yoga, and the Martial Arts—the Core of any Successful Fitness or Sports Program

The visual imagery exercises also introduce you to experiential anatomy. You learn how your body works. Imagery builds the intensity and promotes the safety of every movement. They are an easy, fun way to provide you with the motivation to stay fit.

SUCCESS ▶

A variation of an exercise to help you change your body, and achieve your fitness goals

THE EXTRA EDGE ▶

Highlights an important movement concept to learn how your body works to get results

HOW IT HELPS ▶

Your benefits from an bxercise

Chart Your Progress

THE VISUAL IMAGERY GUIDE

THE VISUAL IMAGERY EXERCISES:

1. Clarify the Alignment, Breathing, and Centering Guiding Principles

2. Enhance your Mind-Body Connection

3. Improve Concentration and Focus

4. Assist in the Control and Execution of a Movement

5. Promote Precision and Attention to the Details of a Movement

6. Balance Relaxation with Muscular Power

7. Emphasize Fluid, Graceful Movements

SUCCESS

THE EXTRA EDGE

HOW IT HELPS

SAFETY

TEACHING TIPS

FITNESS LEVELS

BASIC
INTERMEDIATE
ADVANCED

**THE PRINCIPLES
OF MOVEMENT –
ABCs**

*Alignment • Breathing
Centering and Core Stability*

◀ **SAFETY**
Precautions

◀ **FITNESS LEVELS**

◀ **PRINCIPLES
OF MOVEMENT**

*A reminder to
practice your
alignment,
breathing, and
centering during
an exercise*

YOUR NEEDS

This book is a practical manual containing a comprehensive fitness and stress management program. Depending on your needs, this book offers you a "menu" of choices like at a spa—strength, flexibility, alignment, and breathing exercises—as well as massage, body maintenance routines, and sports conditioning. All of the exercises reinforce important **principles of movement**. The exercises in Part 1 were designed for integration into your everyday activities. The routine practice of them enhances your results in your **Stretching, Pilates, and Sports Mat Programs** in Part 2.

The Basics

VISUAL IMAGERY

The first five chapters contain the basics of the program. How to utilize visual imagery is introduced in Chapter One. This book is written from the standpoint of visualization to integrate the mind and body for success in all the exercises. Empowering exercises are combined with anatomy-based visual imagery. You learn how to access the *power of your mind* through visualization to maintain a healthy, fit, stress-free lifestyle. Like the saying goes, "You can do anything you put your mind to."

Chapter Two introduces you to the essential alignment, breathing, and centering guiding principles.

ALIGNMENT

Alignment techniques presented in Chapter Three organize your skeletal structure. When your bones are in the right place you use the right muscles.

BREATHING AND CENTERING

Chapters Four and Five teach you how to use two completely opposite kinds of breathing patterns to develop either flexibility or strength.

DEEP RELAXATION BREATHING

In Chapter Four you will experience yoga-like breathing. The **Three-Dimensional Breathing Exercise** is a form of deep relaxation breathing. Incorporate it into your stretching program, Desk Freedom exercises, mat workouts, and your daily activities to calm your mind, relax or energize your body.

CENTERED BREATHING FOR EXERCISE AND LIFE

In Chapter Five you will experience a breathing pattern used in Pilates known as ribcage or dynamic breathing. It is distinct from that used in yoga.

The Foundation Exercise helps you to practice this breathing pattern to strengthen your core. The aim is to keep your abdominal and spinal muscles engaged while your ribcage expands as you *inhale*. As you *exhale* the ribcage contracts down towards the waist and involves the deep pelvic muscles.

It is a good idea to warm up with **The Foundation Exercise**. This connects the mind to the body. Your abdominal muscles are warmed up and ready to do the job of guiding every movement. This provides essential stability for movement and energizes the body. **The Foundation Exercise** *is also designed for everyday life. It can be done standing, sitting, lying down, and walking.* You can *power up your core* anytime, anywhere. Everyday tasks such as mowing the lawn, doing house work, carrying groceries, or children become easier to perform with a strong core.

The dynamic breathing also allows you to achieve an exercise rhythm. Use it throughout the **Desk Freedom, Basic Pilates,** and **Sports Mat Programs** for the precise performance of each movement.

This book contains over 70 exercises grouped into categories such as flexibility, strength, and body-maintenance routines. *All* of the exercises focus on Alignment, Breathing, and Centering. These are the key ingredients for success in Pilates, sports, dance, martial arts, yoga, fitness

THREE-DIMENSIONAL BREATHING EXERCISE

See Page 74

FOUNDATION EXERCISE

See Page 83

regimens, and stress management.

The Desk Freedom Exercises focus on these guiding principles of Pilates for your office. Body-maintenance routines such as the **Amazing Sock Ball** and **The Athletic Foot** reduce stress and promote well being. You can practice the mat work at home. Those already doing Pilates can add the **Sports Mat Exercises** to their program. They will help you attain more results through mastering new fitness skills.

COMFORTABLE ENVIRONMENT

You will need an area where you can lie down with enough room to move freely. Lying on a firm, cushioned mat will help support the body. It should be thicker than a yoga mat. If it is too spongy it could make balance difficult. A thick supportive mat will also protect your spine. A specialized Pilates mat is ideal. You may also wish to place your head on a small towel or pillow. The area you choose should be free of distractions such as the phone or television.

CLOTHING

Wear comfortable, loose-fitting clothing that does not restrict your movement. It is preferable to practice with bare feet.

MUSIC

You may prefer to exercise to music. Choose music that helps you focus the mind and body on your workout. Music creates a certain atmosphere. It allows you to turn your attention inward and listen to the rhythm of your own breathing.

WATER

Keep hydrating throughout your exercise sessions. Remember healthy eating, rest and aerobic conditioning such as walking bring about permanent positive changes to your body shape, level of fitness, and general well-being.

CREATE A FITNESS ROUTINE

Aim to practice parts of the program daily. These exercises make that practical because they can be done with any everyday activity. Do more of the program when time permits. It is important to maintain consistency for safety and results.

DESK FREEDOM

See Page 102

AMAZING SOCK BALL

See Page 117

THE ATHLETIC FOOT

See Page 119

SPORTS MAT PROGRAM

See Page 173

Fitness Routines Tailored to Fit Into Your Lifestyle

DAILY CHORES AND ERRANDS: 5 TO 15 MINUTES

ON THE RUN: 5 TO 15 MINUTES

REJUVENATION AT HOME: 5 TO 15 MINUTES

STRETCHING AT HOME: 5 TO 15 MINUTES

AT-HOME STRETCH AND CORE STRENGTH: 20-MINUTE PROGRAM

AT-HOME BODY BUILD: 20-MINUTE PROGRAM

THE PRINCIPLES OF MOVEMENT – ABCs

Alignment • Breathing Centering and Core Stability

AT-HOME STRETCH AND STRENGTH: 30 MINUTES TO ONE-HOUR PROGRAM

AT-HOME CONDITIONING: 30-MINUTES TO ONE-HOUR PROGRAM

AT-HOME POWER UP: THIRTY-MINUTES TO ONE-HOUR PROGRAM

THE PRINCIPLES OF MOVEMENT – ABCs

Alignment • Breathing Centering and Core Stability

STANDING ACTIVITIES FOR YOUR ABCs

RELIEF AFTER STANDING ALL DAY

- The Foundation Exercise — PAGE 83
- Three-Dimensional Breathing — PAGE 74
- Five-Minute Foot Massage — PAGE 121
- Foot Fan and Roots — PAGE 124
- The Amazing Sock Ball Massage — PAGE 117
- Stretching is the Key to Youth — PAGE 131
- Basic Pilates Mat or
  Sports Mat Program — PAGE 147/173

SITTING ACTIVITIES

- The Foundation Exercise — PAGE 83
- Three-Dimensional Breathing — PAGE 74
- Desk Freedom Exercises — PAGE 102
- The Amazing Sock Ball Massage — PAGE 117
- Sit Up and Take Notice — PAGE 43
- Pelvis as a Fish Bowl — PAGE 56

RELIEF AFTER SITTING ALL DAY

- The Foundation Exercise — PAGE 83
- Three-Dimensional Breathing — PAGE 74
- Stretching is the Key to Youth — PAGE 131
- The Amazing Sock Ball Massage — PAGE 117
- Basic Pilates Mat or
  Sports Mat Program — PAGE 147/173

WATCHING TELEVISION

- The Amazing Sock Ball Massage — PAGE 117
- Five-Minute Foot Massage, Foot Fan, and Roots — PAGE 121
- The Foundation Exercise — PAGE 83
- Vertical, Horizontal, Sagittal, and Three-Dimensional Breathing — PAGE 69
- The Desk Freedom Exercises — PAGE 102

**THE PRINCIPLES
OF MOVEMENT –
ABCs**

*Alignment • Breathing
Centering and Core Stability*

WAITING AND LONG LINES

For Standing and Sitting:

For Sitting only:

ROAD WARRIOR TRAVEL FORMULA

AIRPLANE... TO REDUCE JETLAG AND ARRIVE STRESS-FREE

MORNING WAKE UP

DESK FREEDOM SYSTEM

RELAXING BEDTIME PROGRAM

DYNAMIC ENERGIZING PROGRAM

POSTURE PROGRAM

LIVING YOUNGER

PERFORMING ARTS PROGRAM

Actors, Opera Singers, Singers, Musicians, and Performers

SPORTS CONDITIONING ENHANCER FOR ATHLETES AND COACHES

Running, Cycling, Tennis, Golf, Gymnastics, Skating, Hockey, Basketball, Football, Baseball, Soccer, Rugby, Martial Arts, Track and Field, Skiing, Snowboarding, Skateboarding, Swimming, Diving, Surfing, Volleyball, Wrestling, Weight Training, Bodybuilding, Racquetball, Boxing, Rock Climbing, and Equestrian Events.

DYNAMIC DANCE METHOD

Ballet, Jazz, Modern Dance, Ballroom, Tango, and Broadway Dancers, as well as Dance Teachers

THE LIFE EXTENSION SYSTEM
Balance, Vitality, Longevity
Stress Management and Healing Program

*Fitness Participants, Physical Therapists, Movement
Therapists, Occupational Therapists, Caregivers,
Doctors, and Nurses*

EVERYDAY PILATES: THE ABCs

ALIGNMENT EXERCISES:

BREATHING EXERCISES:

CENTERING EXERCISES:

*Also use your ABCs with The Desk Freedom
Exercises, The Amazing Sock Ball Massage,
Roots, and Foot Fan.*

CREATE YOUR OWN PROGRAM

- You Know Best what your Body Needs

Part One

The Essential ABC's for Fitness, Sports, and Everyday Activities

Practice while:

Sitting at your desk or talking on the phone, even watching television.

Standing in a line, shopping, socializing, or playing in the park.

Lying down at home in the morning, before dinner, or on the floor with the kids.

Walking to do your errands, chores, or traveling to any destination...

*Implement these exercises directly into sports, dance,
yoga, martial arts, and gym workouts.*

Chapter One

Visual Imagery is the Key to Success

Remember when you let your imagination run wild as a child? That is what it's like to play with visual images. It is a fun and creative way to change your body. The more dramatically you paint a picture of a visual image in your mind's eye the more complete the results. By using your mind you can develop your body!

This program is for the graceful dancer or athlete within you. Somewhere inside each of us is a performer. A child repeats insistently, "Look at me, look at me!" And to promote their health and fitness, everyone has the ability to tap into their imagination. This book adds visual imagery to *each* exercise. This way fitness becomes fun—never boring—and an outlet for your own creative expression.

Visual imagery is the use of a *mental picture* to accomplish physical tasks. Visualization is an essential element of a good Pilates session. *Every* movement in Pilates engages the mind. You can discover the amazing potential of your body through the use of visual imagery.

Routinely practice these visual imagery exercises with a strong personal desire, intention, patience, and curiosity and you *will* transform your body. Give the exercises your complete attention and let all your other concerns of the day fall

MENTAL PICTURE

Every movement in Pilates engages the mind, and this also unlocks the potential of your body

away. Look at your workouts as an adventure. Explore your body through the power of your mind. You will discover that the body *can* and *does* heal and replenish itself each day.

We think that small aches and pains are a normal part of our lives. But we do not have to suffer from these minor ailments. The body actually wants to function at peak performance. It in fact craves equilibrium, wholeness, and health. The amazing systems of the body operate all day long as a natural pharmacy healing and repairing itself.

This program helps you become aware of new strategies for healthier living. The more energy you invest into taking care of yourself in your younger years, the more it benefits you later. It is never too late to begin a fitness program. The simple preventative measures outlined in this program can make an enormous difference in your health. Joseph Pilates said, "Physical fitness is the first requisite of happiness. In order to achieve happiness, it is imperative to gain mastery of your body. If at the age of 30 you are stiff and out of shape you are old. If at 60 you are supple and strong then you are young."

VISUALIZATION AND IMAGERY TO ACCESS THE MIND-BODY CONNECTION

Visualization and imagery are creative ways to harness the power of the mind-body connection. Visual imagery helps you attain goals: It improves your posture, tones your body, builds athletic skills, and promotes creative expression, health, and healing.

How do visualization and imagery relate to the mind-body connection? *Visualization* involves a thought or what you "see" in the mind's eye. *Imagery* involves the body or what you "feel" with one or all of your senses. Visual imagery is a combination of the two. It requires both *concentration* and *feeling* the sensations in your body. For example, you will find that when you pay attention to how you perform a movement like the **Sit Up and Take Notice** exercise in the next chapter, you connect your mind to your body. A startling thing happens—you improve your posture, which relaxes your muscles *and* calms your mind.

SIT UP AND TAKE NOTICE

See Page 43

These exercises help you focus the power of the imagination to stimulate your innate healing abilities. Creative visualization is a positive way to alleviate worry, fear, or nagging negative thoughts that slip into your consciousness. You are too busy painting a picture in your mind—an image that you can see, smell, taste, hear, or feel, to think of anything else.

Do an experiment. Spend a day using these "instant exercises." Repeat them often throughout the course of your day. Give the imagery work your undivided attention. Increased energy and relaxation are just some of the results you will experience. To change thoughts, feelings, and physiology, you are harnessing the power of creative visualization.

Chapter Two

The Essential ABC
Principles of Movement

ALIGNMENT, BREATHING, AND CENTERING

This is a book to be DONE, not merely read. When you *become* the text and images, you experience your own anatomy. You learn to listen to your body. This heightened awareness of bones, joints, muscles, and breathing lowers your stress levels. You don't need special equipment for this program. With machines, it's easy to be thinking about something other than your workout. Fitness can be achieved with just your own body and intent. For example, a dancer is lean, sleek, and efficient through training that emphasizes proper form and precision. Not having equipment to control helps you focus on core strength and stabilization. When you know how to use your body as a weight, you don't need a gym; you always have a workout with you. The **ABCs** for stress management and fitness lie within your own mind-body connection. But it is helpful to have motivation. The **Alignment, Breathing, and Centering** tech-

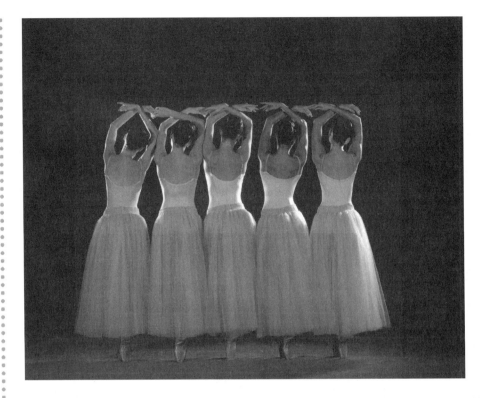

A dancer is lean, sleek, and efficient through training that emphasizes proper form and precision.

George Balanchine's*
SERENADE, Miami City Ballet

Photograph:
© Steven Caras, 2005

*Balanchine is a registered trademark of The George Balanchine Trust

THE PRINCIPLES OF MOVEMENT – ABCs
Alignment • Breathing Centering and Core Stability

niques cover that. They help you start, stick to a plan, and make it fun and safe. Recently a friend learned how easy this portable fitness program could be.

Our morning flight began with my friend MG asking me to teach her this fitness program for people on the go. On take-off she inconspicuously tipped her "Pelvis as a Fish Bowl" and grounded her feet in the center of her "Compass." "The Three- Dimensional Breathing Exercise" softened her facial expression while her butter-like body melted further into the seat. Her cheeks became rosy and she broke into a sweat after a few rounds of "The Foundation Exercise" causing her to strip down. Unlike the other passengers craving a second cup of coffee for the wake up jolt, MG's muscles were experiencing a powerful tune-up fueled by her breathing. By the time I'd introduced her to the pleasures of "The Amazing Sock Ball Massage," she was completely sold. Headset blasting, she was blissfully unaware of her escalating "oohs" and "aahs." Her groans were increasing in volume as the tension in her muscles was being released. In fact, one curious passenger finally remarked, "I'll have what she's having." I talked her through a simple exercise. She easily began to learn how to get fit while on the go.

MG practically bounced off of the plane ready to tackle the hectic day before us. MG said, "This is how I feel after both a great fitness class and a soothing spa treatment—energized yet loose!" MG now knows how to *get fit and live fit*. So can you.

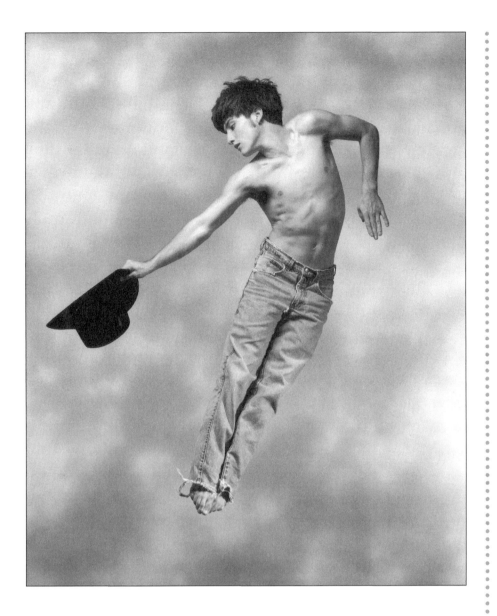

Dancing involves an expressive heart, supple muscles, and an endless drive for precision of the body moving in space.

Dancer/singer/actor
Enrique Brown, 1997

Photograph:
© Steven Caras, 2005

THE EVOLUTION OF THE PRINCIPLES OF MOVEMENT

Joseph Pilates' method was an amalgamation of many different disciplines that he had studied and practiced. These included dance, yoga, the martial arts, and physical therapy. The method emphasizes the *principles of movement* present in all of these disciplines. Joseph worked extensively with dancers to improve their level of performance or rehabilitate them from an injury emphasizing his multi-disciplined approach.

Dancers, martial artists, yoga practitioners, and athletes know that they must analyze movement fundamentals. The guiding principles are necessary for mastering a skill, preventing injury, and exploring movement possibilities. Dance is an art form in which these **Alignment, Breathing and Centering movement principles** are used to achieve artistry and grace. You have seen the beauty of a dancers' body in motion.

37

It is a symphony of suppleness and power.

Dancing involves an expressive heart, supple muscles, and an endless drive for precision of the body moving in space. On stage, there are mystical moments of illumination. A cocoon of concentration envelops you. Your focus turns inward as the body gains momentum. Hard edges vanish leaving only the flow of movement. You are connected to the other dancers by invisible bands of energy. There is an excitement when you push the body beyond its perceived limits. An intimate exchange emerges between the dancer and the audience. The reward is the joy you feel at the end of a performance.

Our Senses

The **ABCs** will teach you that there are these same exhilarating kinesthetic moments within fitness regimens, Pilates, sports, yoga, martial arts, and everyday life. We relate to our world through physical motion and sensory awareness. Children demonstrate this attention to their senses through a natural movement repertoire. In just a few minutes they can run, turn, and fall. They perform all this simply and with complete abandon. Olympic athletes share a child's range of motion and grace, with an adults' strength and mind-body connection.

You can re-discover or enhance this natural grace and flexibility in your own body using the **ABC** exercises. Imagery helps you "fine tune" your senses to a particular exercise. The heart, lungs, and muscles become more alive. A feeling of fitness comes from the inside. When you focus on the quality of an exercise through the use of the **ABCs**, you can change your body. *The basic principles are not separate and distinct. The principles work together to create intelligent, safe, and effective exercise.* The principles teach you how your body functions. By increasing your body awareness you achieve physical skills, mind-body control, and get results.

How the ABCs Help You

Shoulder Blade, Arm, Finger Tip is an **Alignment exercise** located in Chapter Three. It relieves tight neck, shoulder, and upper back muscles. This exercise helps the body operate with more ease of motion in all of your fitness, sports, and daily activities.

The Three-Dimensional Breathing Exercise contained in Chapter Four, focuses on your **Breathing** to calm your mind and create a healthier body. This dynamic breathing pattern replenishes your respiratory system.

The Foundation Exercise helps you to establish a strong body **Core** in Chapter Five. This is how your new inner fitness, grace, and supple muscles will be built. Your **Core** involves your abdominal,

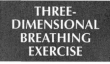

SHOULDER BLADE, ARM, FINGER TIP

See Page 46

THREE-DIMENSIONAL BREATHING EXERCISE

See Page 74

FOUNDATION EXERCISE

See Page 83

back, and buttock muscles. When you train them effectively your body works like a well-oiled machine. **The Foundation Exercise** activates the deep abdominal muscles. This contraction increases the circulation of blood and oxygen to the organs that lie beneath the abdominal wall.

THE ABCs ARE SUPPLEMENTS FOR STRESS-FREE LIVING

Alignment, Breathing, and Centering is not only essential for every efficient dance, sport, and fitness movement. They are also some of the *key ingredients* for increasing your energy level, which can lead to an acceleration of the body's natural healing process after an injury or illness. The same **ABCs** that help a dancer appear ethereal can be used to assist you in elevating your energy to re-establish body harmony.

You can build your energy level through **Breathing** and/or involving your **Core** abdominal muscles. This is accomplished by giving your respiratory system and internal organs additional blood and oxygen. Breathing exercises balance and calm your nervous system. The exercises provide you with ways of working *with* your body for efficiency of motion and better health. You gain more control over your own fitness levels because these powerful **ABCs** boost your immune system.

These healing tools are helpful not only when the body is stressed or out of balance. Add them to this fitness program, sports, walking, weight lifting, or even standing in a post office line for better results.

Never underestimate the seemingly subtle use of these **Alignment, Breathing, and Centering** visual images.

- **Alignment** exercises line-up the bones reinforcing ease and efficiency of motion for the joints and muscles.
- **Breathing** exercises nourish the muscles.
- **Core** abdominal muscle contractions replenish the organs.

This relationship between **Alignment, Breathing, and Centering** is empowering. The most extreme example I encountered occurred while working in an aquatic therapy session with a man who was paralyzed. Despite years of therapy he had never been exposed to the notion of **Breathing** and **Centering**. Once he grasped these principles, he discovered that he could, in fact, move certain parts of his body. By using these techniques he was able to inwardly shape his abdominal muscles. By activating and controlling his breathing, his organs received a deep internal massage.

DANCE AND PILATES CELEBRATE LIFE

The time-honored history of dance celebrates life. Primitive man

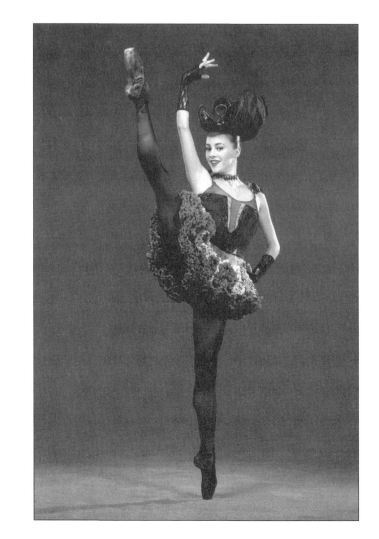

danced around the fire for healing and to mark ritualistic rites of passage. In 1661, the first ballet school was established, eventually giving rise to the modern dance of today.

Dancing, as well as Pilates, encourages discipline, patience, balance, overall vitality, beauty, and creative expression within our lives. These visual imagery exercises promote the artistry, inspiration, and joy of moving. All levels of fitness participants can make important physical changes and have a lot of fun in the process. These **ABC** exercises will help you attain peak performance in fitness, Pilates, sports, dance, yoga, the martial arts, as well as life.

Chapter Three

Alignment is Alive

We pay little or no attention to our body alignment and its relationship to earth's gravitational forces. Yet we feel considerably less stressed when we experience our body moving as an efficient unit through space. Gravity is having an affect on us with every move we make. Even when the body seems very still, there are subtle shifts of weight. Each of these small adjustments relate to the entire body. This is similar to a pebble being thrown into a body of water—it creates a ripple affect. Your body's alignment is never static. The exercises in this chapter will make your body feel like it is grooving with gravity. You will experience that your alignment is alive.

MISALIGNMENTS

Misalignments throw off our body's balanced relationship to gravity. We have all felt our shoulders tense and rise up to our ears. Or we notice that our shoulders are caved inward and downward toward our navel. This round shoulder posture cuts off the air to our lungs. They get scrunched. Stagnant air sits at the base of our lungs. These poor postural habits can contribute to a general feeling of malaise. Good posture can promote confidence, balance, harmony, and better breathing habits. Maintaining an efficient alignment of our skeleton can improve muscle function and range of motion.

YOUR SKELETON

Alignment starts from your skeletal structure. The following alignment exercises will help you find and keep the natural sequence of your skeleton. Place your bones in the right place and you work the right muscles. In the mind-body visual imagery exercises you will primarily experience the arrangement of your bones.

THE USE OF VISUAL IMAGERY

Visual imagery improves your alignment. Imagery is a kind of shortcut to experiencing the mind-body connection. It promotes an awareness and understanding of how your body works. Using imagery will create a new sense of comfort within your body.

Try the following images as you read them. As your body re-aligns itself, your breathing deepens, and you feel relaxed and energized.

VISUAL IMAGERY

A shortcut to the mind-body connection that helps promote an awareness and understanding of your body

THE SIT UP AND TAKE NOTICE EXERCISE

Perform frequently while sitting anytime, anywhere
— at your desk, watching TV, or on an airplane.

Preparation for The Sit Up and Take Notice Exercise

Start with the shoulders and neck. This is where most of us have muscular tension.

1. Lift your shoulders way up toward your ears. Then drop them down. *Scrunch your shoulders up several times.* Add plenty of muscular tension. Relax them back down. Are you breathing deeper as you loosen up your muscles?

2. Sit tall, perched on top of your sit-bones. These are the bones you sit on. They are located at the base of your pelvis. Find them by rocking side to side.

3. Like building blocks—stack your hips, ribs, chest and head on top of each other.

Start The Sit Up and Take Notice Exercise

THE VISUAL IMAGERY GUIDE

1. Picture your shoulder girdle as a shirt. Visualize it hung wide on a clothesline **(FIGURE 3-1)**. The shoulder girdle consists of the region surrounding the collarbone and shoulder blades. Your collarbone is located in the front of your upper body, at the neckline. Your shoulder blades are at each side of your upper back.

2. Gently draw your shoulders backwards.

3. Spread your collarbone wide to the "east and west coasts." *Take several slow, deep, even, and tranquil breaths.* Visualize your inhales filling an imaginary balloon. The balloon is located in between your shoulder blades. Lengthen your inhalations as you picture the balloon expanding. Feel your shoulder blades stretching apart like warm taffy.

4. Imagine your shoulder girdle sliding like molasses into your ribcage.

5. Drop and melt your armpits into the earth.

6. Sense your ribs oozing into your hips like molten lava.

7. Feel your hips melting into your feet like warm butter.

8. Picture your feet sinking deep into the earth growing roots that intertwine and grab onto the earth. **(FIGURE 3-1)**

9. *Now, gently lengthen your body upwards in the opposite direction.* Picture the top of your ears stretching up to reach for the stars.

10. Tighten your abdominal muscles. Picture a zipper for your abdominal muscles. See the zipper closing up your stomach muscles, beginning from your pubic bone and ending at your ribs. **(FIGURE 3-1)** Exhale with force. This helps you contract your stomach muscles in toward your spine. *Try this several times.*

11. Squeeze your buttock muscles and press your inner thighs together. Notice how this helps you to tighten your stomach muscles even more.

Repeat this exercise several times.

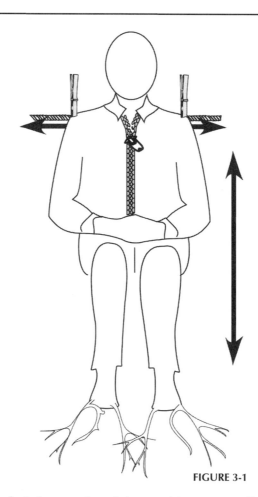

FIGURE 3-1

Do you feel the weight of the world coming off of your shoulders? *Take a few slow, relaxing inhales and exhales.* Enjoy this new sense of freedom in your upper body. *Try lifting your shoulders up high. Now let them go.* Do you feel lighter? You have just experienced the power of using visual imagery to connect your mind to your body.

Take frequent breaks from sitting for long periods of time with the **Sit Up and Take Notice Exercise** for improved health.

THE EXTRA EDGE

FOR THE SIT UP AND TAKE NOTICE EXERCISE

To Highlight the Pilates Principle of Oppositional Lengthening

Oppositional lengthening is an important Pilates technique. It involves the use of lengthening the body in opposite directions. During **The Sit Up and Take Notice Exercise**, parts of your body are connecting into the earth (toward your feet), while other muscles lengthen away in the opposite direction (toward your head). This stretches your body and decompresses your spine.

- Good posture facilitates your ability to contract your core. Oppositional lengthening helps you activate the stabilizing muscles of your trunk, particularly the abdominal muscles.

*Now try **Sit Up and Take Notice** again pressing your feet down while sitting taller. Use the concept of oppositional lengthening by visualizing your body gently stretching apart like a rubber band.* The legs and head lengthen away from the trunk. This promotes the engagement of your core trunk stabilizers toward the central axis within the body.

- You will discover throughout all of your exercises that your center abdominal area is not something you "grab onto" to hold a position. Instead, centering involves an ongoing interchange of motion from the abdominal muscles to the limbs and back again.

OPPOSITIONAL LENGTHENING

Oppositional lengthening improves misalignments and muscular imbalances. It increases the resistance of movements to tone your body.

HOW IT HELPS

- **The Sit Up and Take Notice Exercise** corrects trunk alignment and enhances good posture.

- **Sit Up and Take Notice** helps to lengthen and decompress your spine. The top of your head stretches vertically away from your tailbone. When you lift your head—which weighs approximately 11-13 pounds—gently towards the sky, your body feels lighter. Your head is aligned on top of your spine. The head does not fall forward taking your shoulders with it.

- Your upper trunk is horizontally wider. This makes more room for the lobes of your lungs. It allows you to take deeper breaths. This enhances the health of your respiratory system. Oxygen creates energy for our cells, even our brain cells. Therefore by improving our posture we have better concentration and more physical energy.

- The shoulders slide down away form your ears. Your neck and shoulder muscles have more room to relax.

- This is an excellent exercise for the office, traveling on a plane, or anywhere.

THE SHOULDER BLADE, ARM, FINGER TIP EXERCISE

Perform daily while standing, sitting, walking, and during athletics, dance, yoga, and the martial arts...

Preparation for The Shoulder Blade, Arm, Finger Tip Exercise

Exaggerate the Opposite of The Shoulder Blade, Arm, Finger Tip Exercise. Sit or stand.

1. *Lift your arms to your sides at shoulder level. Then continue lifting them overhead, like a diver.* **(FIGURE 3-2)**

2. Exaggerate this movement. Hike your shoulders up toward your ears. Close off the empty space between your arms and your head. Lifting your arms this high creates a lot of unnecessary tension. You do not need to lift the shoulder girdle up when the arms rise.

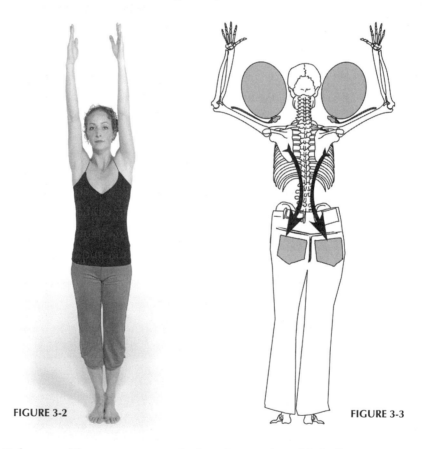

FIGURE 3-2

FIGURE 3-3

Before you lift your arms up again, imagine you have big balloons next to your ears. **(FIGURE 3-3)**

Try it. Notice, you did not elevate your shoulders at all. Your arms stayed several inches away from your head to make room for the balloons. This visual image reinforces a sense of freedom. Feel your arms float up while your shoulder area relaxes downward toward your back trouser pockets.

THE VISUAL IMAGERY GUIDE

START THE SHOULDER BLADE, ARM, FINGER TIP EXERCISE

Lift your arms sideways and then overhead several times.
Before *you move your arms think of guiding your arm movements from your shoulder blades.* **(SEE FIGURES 3-4 AND 3-5)**

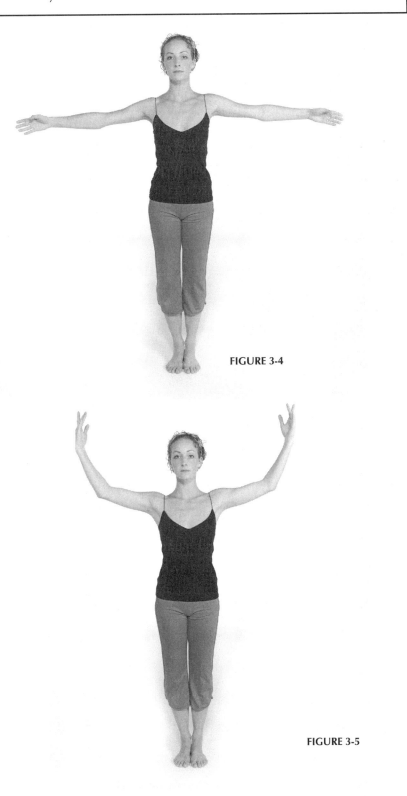

FIGURE 3-4

FIGURE 3-5

Use the following visual imagery to re-pattern the way you lift your arms.

1. When you elevate your arms by first *feeling* a connection to your shoulder blades, the bones of your upper arms can sink downward into the deep sockets of your shoulder joint area. Execute this with minimal muscular tension. The shoulder blades actually move and "float" on the backside of the ribcage.

2. Sense a connection to your collarbone in the front of your body too. Relax the collarbone area each time you lift your arms sideways and then overhead.

3. *Try lifting your arms sideways and then overhead again.* There is an ordered sequence of movement to **The Shoulder Blade, Arm, Finger Tip Exercise.** We are so used to reaching for something from our hands. For more efficient motion begin from the trunk.

     (1) The Shoulder Blades move slightly downward…

     (2) Arms move…

     (3) Finger Tips follow last.

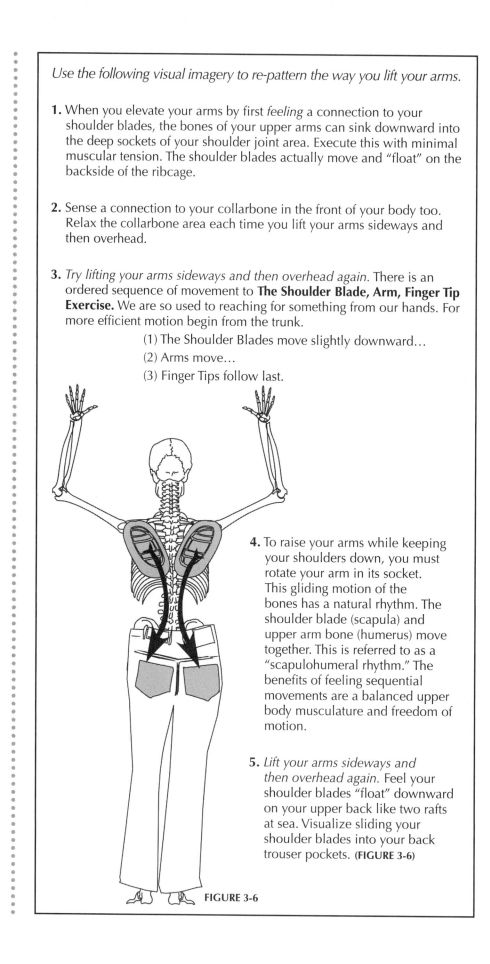

4. To raise your arms while keeping your shoulders down, you must rotate your arm in its socket. This gliding motion of the bones has a natural rhythm. The shoulder blade (scapula) and upper arm bone (humerus) move together. This is referred to as a "scapulohumeral rhythm." The benefits of feeling sequential movements are a balanced upper body musculature and freedom of motion.

5. *Lift your arms sideways and then overhead again.* Feel your shoulder blades "float" downward on your upper back like two rafts at sea. Visualize sliding your shoulder blades into your back trouser pockets. **(FIGURE 3-6)**

FIGURE 3-6

6. *Lift your arms again.* Imagine your shoulder blades as wings. Initiate the movement of your arms as an extension of these wings. Allow the shoulder blades to flatten onto your back.

7. Picture each of your shoulder blades as an oriental fan. The fans spread open as your arms lift. The fans fold and close as your arms lower.

Tactile Discovery with a Partner

*The best way to experience **The Shoulder Blade, Arm, Finger Tip Exercise** is with a partner.*

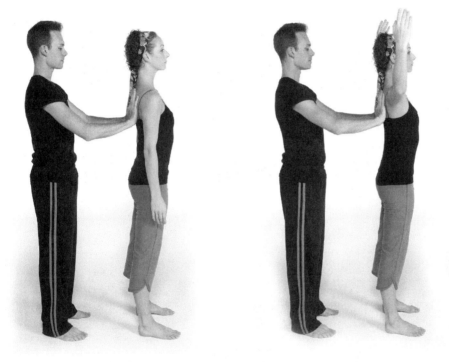

FIGURE 3-7

FIGURE 3-8

1. Each of you takes a turn. Stand behind your partner. Gently place your hands flat against the shoulder blades of the person in front of you, along their upper back. **(FIGURE 3-7)**

2. *Feel how your partner's shoulder blades move, while they lift their arms overhead and back down several times.* **(FIGURE 3-8)**

You will understand the efficient mechanics of your own body through this tactile input. Also try the incorrect way again. Exaggerate lifting your arms sideways and then overhead like a diver. This partner exercise will surprise you. We all use excess muscular tension in our upper body. Use this new knowledge to assist you in relaxing your shoulder area and neck during all the exercises in the book. Enjoy this sense of freedom in your upper body all day long and during any sport activity.

SUCCESS

For the Shoulder Blade, Arm, Finger Tip Exercise

***Try The Shoulder Blade, Arm, Finger Tip Exercise in front of a mirror.** Lift your arms sideways and then overhead several times.*

1. Initiate your arm movements from your shoulder blades instead of your arms. Look at the difference it makes in the mirror.

2. The shoulders stay down. The arms remain away from the head.

3. The upper body spreads wide apart. This gives the muscles, joints, bones, and lungs extra breathing room.

SUCCESS

Try the Opposite: Finger Tip, Arm, Shoulder Blade

1. *Slowly lift your arms sideways and then overhead several times.*

2. Initiate these arm movements from your fingertips. It feels like the fingers float up as the shoulder blades sink downward. You feel the weight of your shoulder blades and shoulders drop comfortably downward. Think of the fingertips and shoulder blades as counterweights.

THE EXTRA EDGE

For the Shoulder Blade, Arm, Finger Tip Exercise

To Highlight the Pilates Principle of Shoulder Girdle Organization

- The upper trunk muscles connect the arms to the body. This shoulder girdle structure stabilizes the upper body so the arms can move with ease.

- In all Pilates exercises, visualize relaxing the shoulder area. Use the image of sliding your shoulder blades, armpits, collarbone, and ribs downward toward your hips during every mat exercise.

HOW IT HELPS

Shoulder Blade, Arm, Finger Tip is a new way of moving your upper body. Muscular tension that is stored in the upper trunk is diminished. This increases your energy level. The body operates with greater ease and range of motion in your activities.

Most of us overuse our "shoulder shrug" and neck muscles in everyday life. We lift our shoulders to hold the telephone, a book, and a car steering wheel. We also write, lift, carry, and work at a computer with round shoulders. This draws the head forward out of alignment with our spine. This exercise will change incorrect, repeated movements of the upper body. You will stop overworking the upper trapezius muscles with every arm movement. Gently stabilizing the shoulder blades and elongating the neck reduces tension and headaches.

Golfers and tennis players have changed their game using this exercise. They attribute winning championships and golfing their lowest score to discovering it. When you perform this exercise you will be moving your arms from their proper biomechanical source of support—your shoulder girdle area and trunk muscles. Contracting the trunk muscles, especially the abdominals, provides more stability for efficient arm movements. Your trunk muscles are your back, chest, abdominals, and hips. Contract your abdominal muscles and use **Shoulder Blade, Arm, Finger Tip** for increased efficiency of motion during basketball shots, swimming strokes, golf swings, tennis serves, or simply reaching for something high on a shelf.

This exercise will teach you to initiate arm movements from your trunk muscles. Economical movements do not originate from a limb. Centered movements require a continual interchange between the trunk muscles and the limbs. Your body then moves as a more efficient unit through space.

TRUNK MUSCLES

Your back, chest, abdominals, and hips are trunk muscles. This exercise will help reduce tension in your upper trunk muscles and increase your energy levels.

THE COMPASS EXERCISE

Perform daily while standing in a grocery store line, at the bus stop, walking the dog, during Pilates, sports, dance, yoga, martial arts, or any performance activity…

THE VISUAL IMAGERY GUIDE

*Perform this exercise standing. Place your feet slightly apart, directly in line with your hipbones—approximately 12 inches apart. The feet stay flat on the ground during **The Compass Exercise**.*

1. Picture yourself standing on top of a compass. *Shift your body weight several times—to the north, south, east, and west of your compass. Pause at each direction.* Sense how your entire body feels during these weight shifts. **(FIGURE 3-9)**

2. Notice the difference between relaxing and tightening your abdominal muscles while performing **The Compass Exercise.** Contracting the abdominals provides more control, better balance, and overall alignment, as well as supporting your lower back.

3. Exaggerate the shifts of your body weight—forward, backwards, sideways, and to the other side. Try *not* to lift your feet off of the floor.

4. Gradually make the motion of your weight shifts smaller and smaller.

5. End by feeling your body weight evenly distributed on the exact *center* of your compass. Balance equally on the balls and heels of your feet.

SUCCESS

*Try **The Compass Exercise** While Walking*

Walk as naturally as possible. Can you keep your body weight evenly distributed over your feet while you are walking? Try not to shift your weight too far in any direction. Move from one foot to the other staying in the center of your feet—or compass.

Experiment with the following walking and balancing exercise:

• When walking the foot hits the ground heel-first then rolls forward. Pay attention to your weight-bearing leg. *When this foot contacts the ground—pause and balance on one leg. Walk again. Try this several times. Practice stopping the forward momentum of your walk to balance on one leg.* Imagine that the sole of your foot—the heel, either side of your arch, and ball of the foot—is evenly placed upon a compass. Plant yourself firmly into the ground each time you pause.

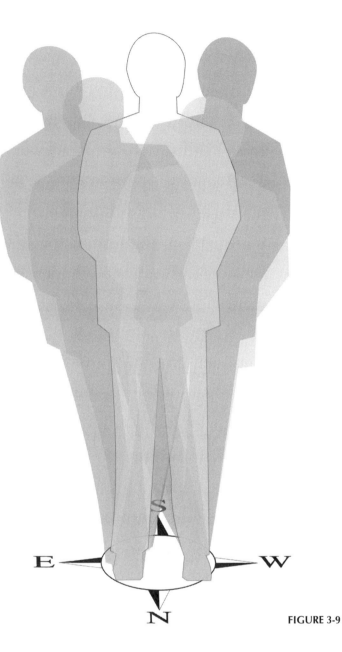

FIGURE 3-9

*Try **The Compass Exercise**, While Standing on One Leg*

(FIGURE 3-10)

1. Stand on one leg only. Lift the other foot off of the floor.

2. Imagine you are standing on a compass. Slightly shift your weight to the north, south, east, and west of the compass.

3. Find the center of the compass.

4. It is helpful to focus on a single spot in front of you.

5. Pay attention to your breathing. We usually hold our breath when we balance. Our muscles become tense and we put the other foot down.

Balance is an important component of fitness. A routine practice of **The Compass Exercise** while standing on one leg makes balancing easy. Relax, play with gravity, and breathe naturally.

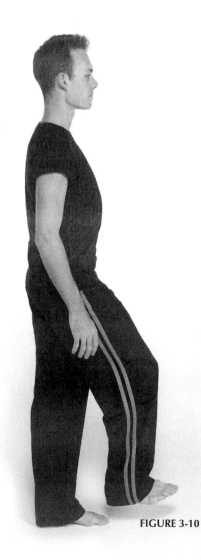

FIGURE 3-10

For The Compass Exercise

To Highlight the Principle of Grounding

Grounding is a term used in the martial arts, dance, and yoga. It refers to the power that emanates from a connection of the body into the ground. Contact and connectedness are maintained by a balanced relationship between the pelvis, feet, and the floor surface. The body's center of gravity is located in the pelvis. Visualize it as a single point in the lower abdomen just below the navel.

Grounding is evident when an opponent throws a martial artist off center. They must regain their balance utilizing a root-like attachment to the floor. Their body must instantly become well aligned, with an equal sense of downward impact into the floor and upward flow away from the floor.

Movement takes on a strong primal quality due to this interchange between the body's weight shifts, gravity, and a deep-rooted connection to the floor. Grounding provides balance and a sense of liquid power during any activity.

Perform **The Compass Exercise** *again*, to feel the relationship between the bones of your feet and the bones of your pelvic floor. Your pelvic floor is located at the base of your pelvis. *The bones of the pelvic floor form a diamond shape between the pubic bone, tailbone, and sit-bones.* Imagine this diamond lifting toward the crown of your head in **The Compass Exercise**. Cough, to feel the muscles of your pelvic floor.

• The *heels* of your feet relate to your *tailbone and sit-bones.*

• The *main arches* of your feet relate to your *sit-bones and pubic bone.*

• The *balls and toes* of your feet relate to your *pubic bone and hipbones.*

HOW IT HELPS

Perform **The Compass Exercise** while standing in long lines. You experience less physical stress by balancing your body's weight evenly over both of your legs. You will be grooving with gravity instead of working against it. This effortless posture lets the bones do the work of holding you up.

The Compass improves the even distribution of the body's weight over the feet. It decreases fatigue and overuse problems. Many misalignments occur from habitually placing all your weight on one leg, leaning into one hip.

Use **The Compass** imagery for balance and weight shifts during all of your activities.

THE PELVIS AS A FISH BOWL EXERCISE

Perform daily while sitting, standing, lying down, walking, and running. It is helpful when lifting heavy objects, or during Pilates, gym workouts, sports, dance, or any activity.

THE VISUAL IMAGERY GUIDE

1. Begin by standing. Contract your stomach muscles. Draw them inward toward your spine. Visualize your navel moving toward your spine.

2. Picture your pelvis as a fish bowl.

3. The rim of the fish bowl is your waistline. *Place your hands on your waist to feel the top of your fish bowl.*

4. *Slightly tip your hips forward.* Visualize water dumping out of the top of your fish bowl in front of you. The lower back arches. The lower spine is in extension. This is called an anterior pelvic tilt. **(FIGURE 3-11. 3-12)**

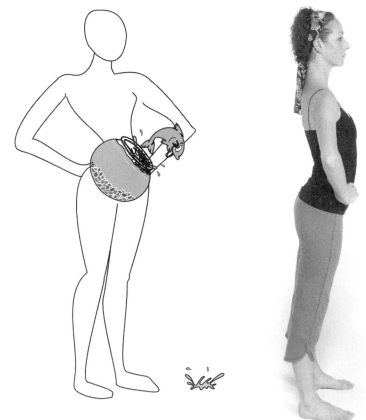

FIGURE 3-11, 3-12: ANTERIOR PELVIC TILT

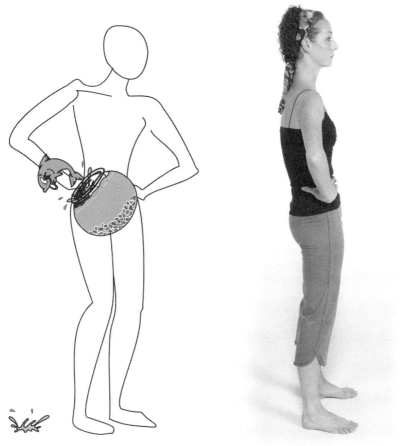

FIGURE 3-13, 3-14: POSTERIOR PELVIC TILT

5. *Tilt your fish bowl backwards.* Slosh water on the floor behind you. The lower back rounds. The lower spine is in flexion. This is called a posterior pelvic tilt. **(FIGURE 3-13, 3-14)**

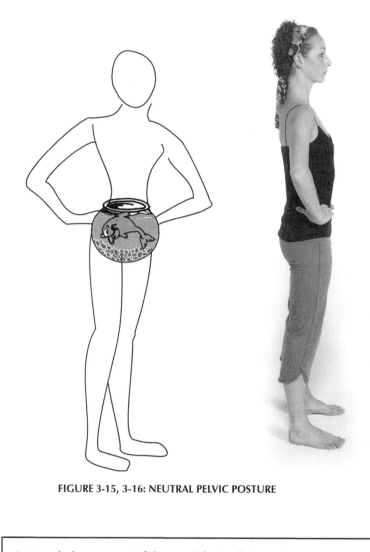

FIGURE 3-15, 3-16: NEUTRAL PELVIC POSTURE

6. *Now balance your **Pelvis as a Fish Bowl**.* Not a drop of water spills. This is called "neutral" pelvic posture. **(FIGURE 3-15, 3-16)** You have a slight natural curve in your lower back. It is important to know where "neutral" is in Pilates and life.

7. *Keep your fish bowl level while you stand up, walk, and sit down.* Did the fish fall out when you were standing, walking, or sitting?

8. Tighten your abdominal muscles while performing **Pelvis as a Fish Bowl**. *Try the exercise again while standing up, walking, and sitting down.* Notice that by contracting your abdominal muscles you take the pressure off of your knees, hip joints, back, and neck. The weight of your body lifts upward out of your legs, away from the floor. You are moving through space from your center abdominal muscles.

THE EXTRA EDGE

For The Pelvis as a Fish Bowl Exercise While Standing

To Highlight the Pilates Principle of a "Neutral" Pelvic Posture

"Neutral" pelvic posture is a fundamental Pilates technique. You just experienced "neutral" pelvic posture in the exercise above. "Neutral" is when your *pelvic fish bowl* is completely balanced. The pelvis does not tip forward or backwards. There are no fish on the floor. You have a slight *natural* curve in your lower back. This precise control of the pelvis and spine is important. It makes movements safe in your fitness programs and in your everyday life.

The Pelvis as a Fish Bowl Exercise *while Lying Down To Find Pilates "Neutral" Pelvic Posture*

Preparation

• Lie down on your back on a mat. Your knees are bent. Your legs are hip width apart. The soles of your feet are flat against the floor. The heels are approximately 12-18 inches from your hips.

• Practice **Pelvis as a Fish Bowl** making your movements gentle and small. Slightly tighten your abdominal muscles toward your spine.

Start
Step One

Curl your lower back by tipping your pelvic fish bowl backwards. Visualize the water spilling out the back of your waistline. Your lower back is gently *resting against the floor*. Your lower back is in flexion with a slight posterior pelvic tilt. **(FIGURE 3-17)**

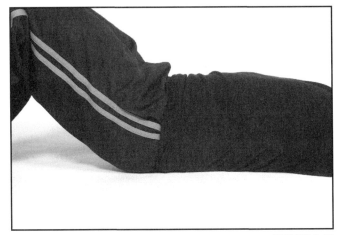

FIGURE 3-17

Step Two

Arch your lower back by tipping your pelvic fish bowl forward. Picture water spilling out of the front of your waistline. Your lower back is slightly arched—*away from the floor*. Your lower back is in extension with a slight anterior pelvic tilt. **(FIGURE 3-18)**

Step Three

1. Now find your **"neutral"** pelvic posture by moving between this **curl** and **arch** position. Make your movements smaller and smaller.

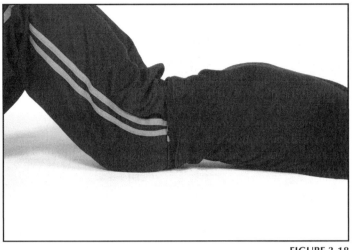

FIGURE 3-18

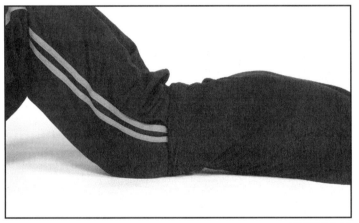

FIGURE 3-19

2. Feel "neutral" as the middle place of balance right in between the curl and arch of your pelvis. (FIGURE 3-19)

3. In "neutral" posture your hipbones and pubic bone are level with each other. They are parallel to the mat. There is a slight *natural* arch in your lower back. You could serve a cup of tea on your pelvis without spilling the tea.

Use "neutral" pelvic posture for all of your exercise programs, including the mat work.

You have experienced how visualization works during the alignment exercises in this chapter. By using your mind you can develop your body. Visual imagery makes the process fun.

In Pilates your mind takes a constant internal "survey" of each part of your body. You develop an inner "detective." Visualize your entire body working as a unit with each repetition of an exercise. Every movement is fresh and never boring.

Movement in Pilates engages the mind. Visualization is essential to a good fitness session. As you practice these exercises during your everyday activities, sports, and mat exercises, paint a vivid picture in your mind of the visual image to attain success. You will be using these mind-body visual imagery alignment exercises to re-pattern inefficient movement habits, acquire new physical skills, and prevent injury.

These alignment exercises reinforce the important Pilates concept of *moving your body as a unit*. The trunk and limbs are integrated within each movement. The following *general bony landmarks* of your entire body are included in the Alignment exercises in this chapter:

1. *The top of your head/tailbone connection* is used in **The Sit Up and Take Notice Exercise** and **The Pelvis as a Fish Bowl Exercise**.
2. Your *heel/sit-bone connection* is used in **The Compass Exercise**.
3. Your *shoulder blade, arm, finger tip connection* is used in the **Shoulder Blade, Arm, Finger Tip Exercise**.

Routine practice of the exercises in this chapter will result in a more balanced total body alignment.

Chapter Four

Three-Dimensional Breathing

Breathing is the bridge between the mind and the body. When the breathing is steady so is the mind. Conscious controlled breathing is an essential part of yoga. Yoga calls it prana, which means life force or energy. Yoga has long recognized that breathing is the main manifestation of prana. It also can be found in air, water, earth, sunshine, and animals.

Many of us breathe shallowly. We barely fill the upper area of the chest with our inhalations. Sometimes we take in only about one-third of the oxygen needed by the lungs. We were designed to be deep abdominal breathers. This is evident in the unrestricted movements of a baby's belly.

How we breathe directly affects our nervous system and therefore our immune system. Breathing is the link to our state of mind. Fear shortens our breathing. When we are stressed it becomes shallow and resides high in the chest. Breathing becomes erratic when we feel anxious. It practically disappears when we concentrate hard.

You can reach the peaceful breathing rhythm of sleep by practicing the **Three-Dimensional Breathing Exercises** in this chapter. Your breathing becomes slow and quiet. You

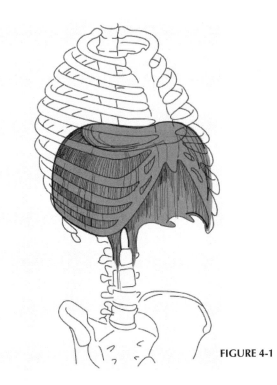

FIGURE 4-1

feel calm. The difference between shallow and deep abdominal breathing is the role of your *diaphragm*. When you pay attention to deep relaxation breathing you can affect this most important and underrated muscle of the body—and your health.

CHANGING YOUR VIEW OF THE WORLD

You can exercise your breathing muscles by understanding how they work. The *diaphragm* connects to the breastbone, the lower ribs, and the lower spine. It serves as a floor for the chest and a ceiling for the stomach.

During an *efficient* inhalation, the *diaphragm* drops down toward the abdomen. The *diaphragm's* down stroke massages the abdominal wall and organs as the chest enlarges.

In order for the *diaphragm* to work properly, the abdominal muscles must relax and slightly expand. If not, the *diaphragm* cannot drop down. The breath stays up in the narrower passages of the chest. Here is where the term shallow chest breathing comes from. Shallow breathing can contribute to lethargy, anxiety, and stress within our lives.

During an *efficient* exhalation, the *diaphragm* will relax and move up into the chest. At this point in the breathing cycle, the *diaphragm* takes on a dome-like shape. It looks like a parachute. **(FIGURE 4-1)** This motion is executed by a gentle tightening of the abdominal wall. The chest relaxes and the ribs press toward the lungs. Deep relaxation breathing promotes calmness, confidence, vitality, and harmony within your life.

DIAPHRAGM

Connects to your breastbone, lower ribs, and lower spine. It is essential for deep breathing.

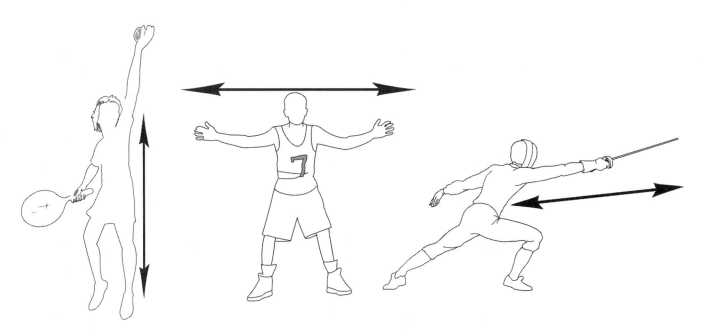

FIGURE 4-2: VERTICAL DIRECTION **FIGURE 4-3: HORIZONTAL DIRECTION** **FIGURE 4-4: SAGGITAL DIRECTION**

The habit of shallow breathing weakens the *diaphragm* muscle and the muscles of the ribs. It deprives the chest and abdominal area of stimulation, which affects digestion and circulation. Stale air remains lodged in the lower lungs. The blood lacks the necessary oxygen and is burdened with toxins.

Joseph Pilates said, "To breathe correctly you must completely exhale and inhale, always trying very hard to 'squeeze' every atom of impure air from your lungs in much the same manner that you would wring every drop of water from a wet cloth."

INTRODUCTION TO THE THREE DIMENSIONS

We are three-dimensional beings living in a three-dimensional world. Our bodies have (vertical) length, (horizontal) width, and (sagittal) depth. These three planes define direction and location for the body.

Complex body movements typically involve movement in all three planes. However, there are movements that emphasize one direction. You can move primarily in the *vertical direction* (up and down) like during a *tennis serve*, the *horizontal direction* (side to side) like a *basketball guard's lateral movements*, and the *sagittal direction* (forward and back) like the *thrust of a sword in fencing*. **(FIGURES 4-2, 4-3, 4-4)**

Moving the body in the vertical plane corresponds to rising and shrinking movements. Moving the body in the horizontal plane involves widening and narrowing movements. Moving the body in the sagittal plane utilizes advancing and retreating movements.

INTRODUCTION TO THREE DIMENSIONAL BREATHING

The **Three-Dimensional Breathing Exercise** is an *ally* for your body's movements. For example, breathing can support the intricate motion of a

OUR THREE DIMENSIONS

Three planes define direction and location for the body: Length (vertical), width (horizontal), and depth (sagittal).

tennis serve. The vertical lift and toss of the ball occurs during a full inhalation. You have heard the powerful groan on the exhalation as the tennis player's racket makes contact with the ball and throughout the downward stroke of the motion. Awareness of your breathing can contribute to the intensity and clarity of the body's three-dimensional movements into the vertical, horizontal, and sagittal directions in space.

The **Three-Dimensional Breathing Exercises** help you access your mind-body connection. You can make it your intention to fill the interior spaces of your body with air. Visual imagery makes it possible to direct your inhalations into one or all three of these directions. With practice you can visualize directing air to the outermost boundaries of your body.

Three-Dimensional Breathing supports our body's multi-directional movements. Your breathing will become more efficient using this form of deep diaphragmatic breathing. You can learn to balance and lengthen the cycle of your inhalations and exhalations.

BREATHING SUCCESS

Perform the breathing exercises in this chapter daily while in any position—sitting, standing, lying down, or walking—anytime, anywhere. It is helpful for stress management, or during this fitness program, stretching, Pilates, sports, yoga, martial arts, dance, gym workouts, rehabilitation, and everyday activities.

- These are **DEEP, SLOW, EVEN, AND TRANQUIL BREATHS.** Imagine your breathing is like the motion of an ocean wave. Inhale, visualizing your breath spreading over the shoreline. Exhale, picturing your breath washing back out with the tide.

- The breathing exercises help your abdominal area expand for a full, deep breath. The belly must move outward for a full volume of air to move into the lungs.

- It is more relaxing to breathe in through the nose and out through the mouth. The nose filters impurities in the air.

- Allow your breathing to flow naturally without force or strain.

- Find a rhythm comfortable for you. This may be about a slow eight count inhale and a slow eight count exhale. Practice over time and you may gradually increase this rhythm to a comfortable fifteen or twenty count inhale, and a fifteen or twenty count exhale.

- Balance the length of your inhalations and exhalations.

- *Relax all the muscles of your body.* Turn your focus inward. Pay attention to your breathing to the exclusion of everything else in your life.

- Practice for only three to five minutes a session.

SAFETY

Discontinue your practice at any sign of strain, tension, or lightheadedness. Working with your breathing takes time, patience, and concentration. Never hold your breath when working with breathing techniques.

THE CONSTRUCTIVE REST POSE

This is an ideal way to begin practicing breathing.
You can relax more readily.

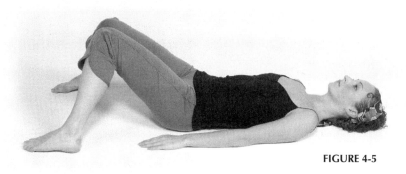

FIGURE 4-5

Prepare for the Breathing Exercises in The Constructive Rest Pose

Wear loose comfortable clothing. Elevate your head slightly with a towel. This lengthens your neck. Your air passages become open for a free exchange of oxygen. Your chin is slightly tipped toward your chest. **(FIGURE 4-5)**

1. Lie on your back with your knees bent. The soles of your feet are on the floor, approximately two feet apart.

2. Allow your knees to meet, creating a teepee shape with your legs. Your bent knees encourage your lower back to lengthen.

3. Your arms are by your sides. Keep your shoulders down away from your ears.

THE VERTICAL BREATHING EXERCISE

Perform daily in any position—sitting, standing, lying down, or walking—anytime, anywhere.

THE VISUAL IMAGERY GUIDE

Vertical Breathing can assist you in becoming a graceful athlete. *Imagine yourself diving, high jumping, or shooting a basketball. Use the following exercise to gain "air time" for these rising and falling movements.*

Remember: these are **deep, slow, even, and tranquil inhalations and exhalations.**

POSITION FOR THE VERTICAL BREATHING EXERCISE

Begin in **The Constructive Rest Pose**. See preparation above for **The Constructive Rest Pose.**

Start

Let your *inhalations* make your body feel *taller*.

1. Picture a LONG SAUSAGE-SHAPED BALLOON inside your body. Visualize filling this balloon with air *up and down, vertically*. See the balloon lengthen and expand on your long, slow inhales. **(FIGURE 4-6)** Envision the balloon shrinking on your exhales.

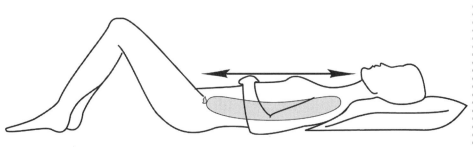

FIGURE 4-6

2. Inhale, imagining the balloon expanding simultaneously from the bottom of your pelvis to the top of your shoulders.

3. Exhale, visualizing the balloon deflating into the center of your body.

4. Inhale, picturing your balloon expanding along the entire length of your spine. Imagine your tailbone lengthening toward your feet, and your head rising. Exhale.

CONSTRUCTIVE REST POSE

See Page 68

5. Inhale, visualizing your tailbone becoming a long dinosaur tail. Exhale.

6. See your head as a helium balloon that floats on top of a long spine while inhaling. Visualize your head soaring away from your spine. Exhale, picturing your balloon deflating.

7. Place one hand high on your chest and the other hand low on your belly. Inhale, feel your hands stretch away from each other. Exhale, while noticing how your hands come closer together. **(FIGURE 4-7)**

Try this several times.

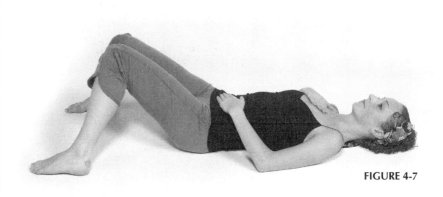

FIGURE 4-7

8. Did you feel your ribcage rise up away from your hips on your inhales? Fill the entire back surfaces of your body with air—lower back, ribcage, and shoulder blades. Does your spine feel longer? Did you feel your hips and head stretch away from one another? Exhale. The bones of your spine stay long while the muscles around them relax.

9. Inhale, directing your breath up and down throughout your entire body like an elevator that moves between the floors. Exhale.

THE HORIZONTAL BREATHING EXERCISE

Perform daily in any position—sitting, standing, lying down, or walking—anytime, anywhere.

THE VISUAL IMAGERY GUIDE

Picture yourself performing lateral movements with athletic grace. See your body move like a basketball guard or speed skater. To produce these widening and narrowing movements, imagine filling your body with air like a bellows, expanding and contracting.

Remember: these are deep, slow, even, and tranquil inhalations and exhalations.

POSITION FOR THE HORIZONTAL BREATHING EXERCISE
Begin in The Constructive Rest Pose.

Start
Let your *inhalations* make your entire trunk feel wide.

1. *Place your hands on either side of your ribcage. Your fingertips are touching.*

2. Inhale slowly and deeply. Your fingertips will move away from each other. **(FIGURE 4-8)**

CONSTRUCTIVE REST POSE

See Page 68

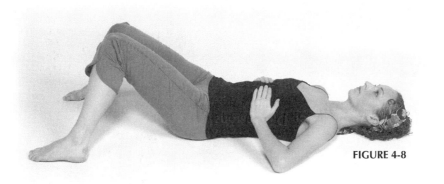

FIGURE 4-8

3. Exhale, and your hands will gradually come back together.

4. Picture a WIDE BALLOON inside your body. Visualize filling this balloon with air *sideways, horizontally.* See the balloon widen on your inhales. Envision the balloon becoming narrow on your exhales. Inhale again. Exaggerate the sideways and backwards expansion of the balloon into your lower ribcage. Exhale, picturing the balloon gradually

collapsing inward toward your breastbone, spine, and navel. This is referred to as "lateral breathing" in Pilates.

5. *Try the* **Horizontal Breathing** *with your hands on your belly several times.*

6. Inhale. Feel your hands widen away from each other. Stretch apart the right and left halves of your body. Exhale, allowing your hands to come back together. This is like the slow motion of an accordion opening and closing. **(FIGURE 4-9)**

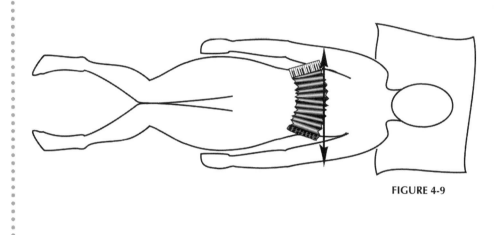

FIGURE 4-9

7. *Place your hands against your hipbones.* Breathe in and out slowly. Did you feel the area around your hipbones open wide on your inhalations?

8. *Place your hands around your waistline.* Slowly expand your waistline with air. Exhale, narrowing your waistline.

9. Picture your ribs and shoulders stretching to touch the wall on the right and left side of the room during your inhales. Exhale. Visualize your inhalations open your armpits like the gills of a fish. Exhale.

10. Inhale, busting every button on your shirt. Exhale.

11. Picture yourself standing inside a doorframe. Direct your intake of air sideways. Imagine that your trunk can thicken and grow sideways until your outer arms, ribs, and hips touch both sides of the doorframe. Exhale.

THE SAGITTAL BREATHING EXERCISE

Perform daily in any position—sitting, standing, lying down, or walking—anytime, anywhere.

THE VISUAL IMAGERY GUIDE

Imagine you are a martial artist, boxer, fencer, or baseball pitcher. Visualize directing your intake of air forward and backwards within your body to support these powerful advancing and retreating movements.

Remember: these are **deep, slow, even, and tranquil inhalations and exhalations**.

Position for The Sagittal Breathing Exercise
Begin in **The Constructive Rest Pose**.

Start

1. Let your *inhalations* make your body feel *thick*.

2. *Place one hand on your belly and your other hand beneath you on your lower back.* Picture a THICK, FAT BALLOON inside your body. Visualize filling this balloon with air *forward and backwards, sagittaly*. Exhale. **(FIGURE 4-10)**

CONSTRUCTIVE REST POSE

See Page 68

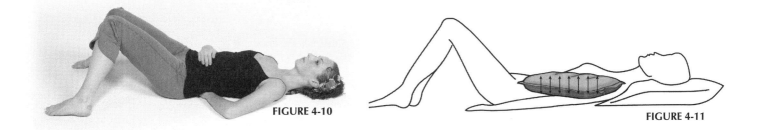

FIGURE 4-10

FIGURE 4-11

3. Inhale again. Feel the balloon thicken. It can simultaneously expand toward the ceiling and into the floor. Exhale, visualizing the balloon flatten like pancake batter across a skillet. Feel the weight of your body sink into the floor during your exhales.

4. Picture your body as a plastic floating raft, gradually being filled with air. The air mattress deflates on your exhales. *Try this several times.* During your inhalations, did you feel your chest, ribs, and belly, stretch up to the ceiling? Simultaneously, did you feel the back surfaces of your body expand into the floor—your shoulder blades, ribcage, and lower back? Exhale. **(FIGURE 4-11)**

5. Imagine a Buddha belly or a billowing sail while breathing in. Exhale.

6. Visualize your body puffing outwards like a pillow during your inhales. The pillow flattens on your exhales.

THE THREE-DIMENSIONAL BREATHING EXERCISE

Perform daily in any position—sitting, standing, lying down, or walking—anytime, anywhere.

THE VISUAL IMAGERY GUIDE

Visualize yourself as a graceful ice skater, gymnast, or dancer. Imagine directing your intake of air in every direction. Fill the interior spaces of your body vertically, horizontally, and sagitally.

*Remember: these are **deep, slow, even, and tranquil inhalations and exhalations.***

Preparation for The Three-Dimensional Breathing Exercise

- Begin in **The Constructive Rest Pose**. You may want to warm up for the **Three-Dimensional Breathing** with the **Vertical, Horizontal, and Sagittal Breathing Exercises** above.

Start

1. Let your inhalations MAKE YOUR BODY FEEL *TALL, WIDE, AND THICK.*

2. Picture a LONG, WIDE, AND THICK BALLOON inside your body. Visualize filling this balloon with air *vertically, horizontally, and sagittaly. Try this several times.*

3. Inhale, imagining your body stretching from the inside outward. See your balloon expand to have length, width, and depth.

4. Exhale, picturing the balloon in your mind's eye shrinking from all three directions. Your balloon deflates into the center of your body. *Take several long, slow, tranquil breaths.*

5. Inhale, envisioning your body as a hot air balloon that you are inflating. Exhale, watching the hot air balloon collapse. Alternate filling your hot air balloon vertically, then horizontally, and finally sagittally during a SINGLE INHALATION. **(FIGURE 4-12)** Exhale.

6. Try mixing up the directions of your single inhale between length, width, and depth. Clearly picture each separate direction in your mind while inhaling. While practicing a single inhalation, say to yourself, "up and down, then side-to-side, and finally forward and backwards". Exhale.

CONSTRUCTIVE
REST POSE

See Page 68

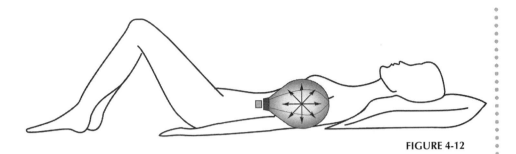

FIGURE 4-12

You have just done "spring cleaning" for your lungs. Do these breathing exercises several times a day for your health. Joseph Pilates said, "Before any real benefit can be derived from physical exercises, one must first learn how to breathe properly. Our very life depends on it."

Pay attention to how the breathing exercises make you feel. Your muscles are deeply relaxed. You have gotten rid of extra muscular tension. Your mind is quiet. You feel calm.

Through practice you will notice improvements in concentration and energy level. You will have better posture because you are more aware of the vertical, horizontal, and sagittal space within and around your body.

THE EXTRA EDGE

TO HIGHLIGHT THE PILATES PRINCIPLE OF "LATERAL BREATHING"

Efficient breathing in Pilates is referred to as "lateral breathing." The emphasis is on the horizontal direction. As you *inhale*, feel your lower ribcage expand sideways and backwards. The muscles in between your individual ribs stretch and widen.

During an efficient *exhalation* in Pilates, the ribcage comes back together and moves down toward the pelvis. This feels like your ribcage is a corset, which cinches together in the front of your body. Try this efficient inhalation and exhalation. It will make you feel refreshed and alive.

In Pilates you need to fill your lungs completely and then wring out every ounce of air. This is a "breath bath" for your cells. It cleans and nourishes your body.

• *The inhalation in Pilates should not just emphasize the lateral direction. The use of* **Three-Dimensional Breathing** *during exercise will help you to breathe along the entire back surfaces of your body—the shoulder blade area, middle, and lower back. It includes directing air under your breastbone and into your armpits.*

• There will be less expansion to the front of the body during the inhalation while performing Pilates movements. This is because the abdominal contraction is always maintained during the inhalation and exhalation of every movement. Avoid breathing high into the chest as this can also involve lifting the shoulders and chest.

In your mat exercises, put your attention on long, slow, and even breaths. Breathe out forcefully while contracting your core trunk muscles. This provides assistance for moving your body with precision into three-dimensional space.

HOW IT HELPS

How The Vertical, Horizontal, Sagittal, and Three-Dimensional Breathing Exercises Help You

- Practicing the **Three-Dimensional Breathing Exercise** provides inward support for the outward directions of your body's movements into space.

- By making more room for air in the body, **Three-Dimensional Breathing** pushes out and filters stagnant air.

- During everyday activities, exercise your breathing muscles for a quick and convenient pick-me-up.

- No fancy equipment is necessary to energize and/or relax your body—just use your **Three-Dimensional Breathing**. Practice breathing in the morning, before sleep, or standing in a long line.

- Controlled breathing enhances your ability to cope with stress. Breathing is directly related to calming the nervous system. The body is refreshed, which in turn calms the mind. Use it during a hectic workday or on a long plane flight.

- This efficient diaphragmatic breathing becomes an inner massage that replenishes your organs.

- These breathing techniques invigorate the muscles of the ribs, diaphragm, and back.

- Exercising your respiratory system improves metabolic and cardiovascular function.

- It increases lung capacity.

- This exercise develops your powers of paying attention to your breathing—which is your most immediate life-sustaining source—so you can affect it. This is breath "insurance" for better concentration, energy levels, sleep patterns, and digestion.

- These breathing exercises are excellent for the warm up, range, and care of the voice of singers, actors, and speakers. It adds authority and calmness to the voice.

- This breathing technique provides inner support for your posture. It relaxes tight muscles along the spine, neck, shoulders, ribcage, and lower back.

- This breathing pattern can prepare the mind for silence in meditation. Many of us find it difficult to meditate. This exercise solves that problem by providing something concrete to focus on.

- Use it in your stretching program to improve your relaxation and range of motion.

- **Three-Dimensional Breathing** enlarges the inner cavities, volumes, or spaces within the body. This provides more core abdominal control for the movements of Pilates. The more air you take in, the more your abdominals can contract during your exhales. It is also essential for other forms of fitness training, sports, and dance.

- Breathing helps coordinate and blend one movement into the next. It supports the pacing and rhythm of your Pilates, sports, and daily movements.

- The breathing techniques provide a physical sense of security, confidence, grounding, vitality, and passion for being alive.

Chapter Five

The Foundation Exercise

PUT YOUR MIND ON YOUR MUSCLES TO FIND THE PILATES POWERHOUSE

Picturing your abdominal muscles during **The Foundation Exercise** is the key to toned, strong stomach muscles. Your center abdominal area is the most essential ingredient for Pilates, and *Functional Fitness* training. Pilates calls your center the Powerhouse. The Powerhouse is located in the middle of the body. It is the area of the trunk between your lower ribs and hips. The **abdominal muscles** form the *foundation* of your body's powerful midsection. The Pilates Powerhouse includes the abdominals, lower back, hips, and buttock muscles. A strong Powerhouse is the foundation for all Pilates exercises.

In Pilates your abdominal muscles become the "steering wheel" for all of your movements. Your breathing is the fuel for firing up and deeply contracting your abdominals. When you strengthen these core muscles of your body, it works like a well-oiled machine. Many of us find it difficult to feel our stomach muscles contract. It is particularly challenging to locate the deep layers of the abdominals. The deepest layers are the most important for Pilates and fitness results. **The Foundation Exercise** helps you master this deep core control through imagery. You first picture the abdominals. Concentration helps you locate them and inwardly shape them. You develop an awareness of degrees of muscular contraction for efficient movement without overusing any muscles.

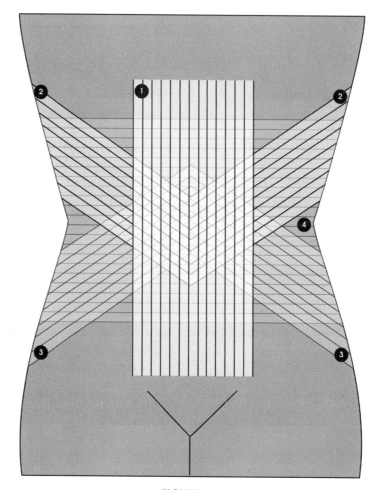

FIGURE 5-1
PICTURE ... YOUR ABDOMINAL MUSCLES AS AN ANATOMICAL GIRDLE:
THE ABDOMINAL MUSCLES ARE MADE UP OF FOUR LAYERS OF
POWERFUL ELASTIC BANDS. THESE MUSCLE FIBERS CRISSCROSS TO
FORM AN ANATOMICAL GIRDLE. THEY LIE ACROSS EACH OTHER AT
VARIOUS ANGLES.

THE FOUNDATION EXERCISE

Pilates was designed to train the *deeper functional muscles* of the body. This emphasis on the smaller, postural muscles provides support for the larger, superficial, structural muscles of the body. *Functional Fitness training is fitness from the inside out.* **The Foundation Exercise** helps you activate the deeper layers of the abdominal muscles, which are responsible for proper breathing, good posture, and organ and spine support.

It is helpful to first *picture* the abdominals to *find* them, and then *feel* them contract. The abdominal muscles are made up of four layers of powerful elastic bands.

These muscle fibers crisscross to form an *anatomical girdle*. They lie across each other at various angles. **(FIGURE 5-1, 5-2)** The abdominal muscles attach to your ribcage and to your pelvis. They provide trunk stability and mobility.

Every Pilates movement emanates from your abdominal muscles. In **The Foundation Exercise,** visual imagery and picturing your anatomy are combined to provide a shortcut to *feel* the deep contraction of your abdominal muscles toward your spine.

This exercise requires concentration. Practice putting your mind on your abdominal muscles and this exercise will become second nature. Mastering this centering technique provides success and safety for all of your exercises, sports, dance, martial arts, and life.

The abdominal muscles contract as a unit to produce movements. Nevertheless, **The Foundation Exercise** uses *visual imagery* to *isolate* each of the four layers of your abdominal muscles groups, step by step.

Picturing the anatomy of the abdominal muscles helps you to tone your stomach area like never before. A strong abdominal core offers limitless reserves of power for any activity. You can reach your full movement potential.

The Four Abdominal Muscle Groups

From the Outermost Layer to the Deepest Layer within the Body

1. Rectus Abdominis
2. External Obliques
3. Internal Obliques
4. The Transversus Abdominis

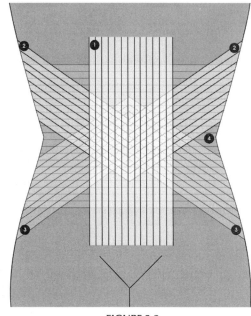

FIGURE 5-2
THE FOUR ABDOMINAL MUSCLE GROUPS

1. The **outermost** *rectus abdominis* muscle fibers run **vertically** *down the entire front of your body's midsection.* The fibers run essentially parallel to each other. You are looking at these muscles when you see a body builder's "six-pack." It is the only layer of abdominals that does not connect to your back. Therefore these outer structural muscles are not as effective for spinal stability, breathing assistance, or organ support as the deeper functional abdominals.

Muscular Lines of Force: The *rectus abdominis* muscles originate at the pubic bone and insert beneath the breastbone. They draw the front of the pelvis **upwards** towards the ribs. **This is why the image of a *jaw closing* is the first step in The Foundation Exercise.**

2. The *external obliques* are the **second** layer of the Pilates Powerhouse. The muscle fibers take on the shape of a fan. They crisscross diagonally with the *internal obliques*, like an X that wraps around the body. These muscles compress the abdomen together and backwards toward the spine, in a sagittal direction. **This is why the image of an *upper corset* is the second step in The Foundation Exercise.** These muscles wrap *from the back of the ribs around to the front and then downward toward the hips.* They cinch the body together like a corset.

Muscular Lines of Force: The *external obliques* originate at the lower eight ribs and insert at the top of the pelvis. When they contract they draw the back of the ribcage to the front, and then down into the hips like a corset.

3. The *internal obliques* are the **third** layer of your abdominals. These muscle fibers cross the midriff in diagonal slants *from the top of the hips,* **up-**

ward *to the lowest part of the ribcage.* **This is why the image of a** *lower girdle* **is the third step in The Foundation Exercise.** The powerful elastic action of these muscles feels like a girdle drawing your abdominal wall in, backwards, and upwards. Imagine these muscles lifting your body up, like the motion of a dancer leaping into the air.

Muscular Lines of Force: The *internal obliques* originate at the pelvic rim and insert on the last four ribs.

4. The *transversus abdominis* is the **fourth** and **deepest** layer closest to your spine. They consist of muscle fibers that contract in a horizontal direction to **encircle** the torso. Engaging these muscles stabilize the spine and pelvis. It is the only abdominal muscle that attaches to your diaphragm and supports healthy breathing. This muscle ideally contracts first in all Pilates movements. It gets very strong. Movements become safe. This deepest layer is responsible for drawing the rest of the belly inward. This is how you achieve a flat tummy. **This is why the two images of** *hug* **and** *navel to your spine* **are the final steps in The Foundation Exercise.**

Muscular Lines of Force: The *transversus abdominis* muscles originate at the pelvic rim and the cartilages of the last six ribs. They insert at the breastbone and pubic bone.

SUCCESS

Simultaneously Engage your Abdominals and the Base of your Pilates Powerhouse During the Five Steps of The Foundation Exercise

The base of your Powerhouse includes your buttocks, pelvic floor, and upper leg muscles. To engage these muscles, squeeze your buttocks and your inner thighs together.

To Prepare for the Five Steps of The Foundation Exercise

1. **NEVER LET YOUR ABDOMINALS RELAX IN BETWEEN THE FIVE STEPS.** Keep inwardly shaping and moving them. BY INCREASING YOUR ABILITY TO *DEEPEN* THE CONTRACTION OF YOUR ABDOMINALS YOU WILL CHANGE THE LOOK OF YOUR STOMACH.

2. Blend one step into the next without relaxing the abdominals. Move slowly in order to feel the abdominals move in deeper and deeper toward your spine during each step of **The Foundation Exercise.**

3. *Keep the abdominals tight during your inhales and exhales.* Lengthen your exhalations and make an outward sound as the air releases. This is when your abdominals move inward. **Feel the power of your breathing and your abdominals working in concert with each other.**

Practice The Five Steps of The Foundation Exercise
Perform daily while in any position, and while walking, running, traveling—anytime, anywhere. It is also essential for any fitness regimen, sport, dance, martial art, yoga, performance activity, and rehabilitation.

PICTURE ... A JAW CLOSING

Position for Step One of The Foundation Exercise. **(FIGURE 5-3)**

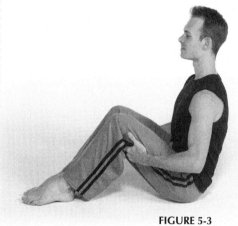

1. Sit on the floor on a mat.

2. Your knees are bent.

3. The soles of your feet are on the floor.

4. Your legs are together.

5. Wrap your hands behind your thighs.

6. Draw your waistline in and up.

FIGURE 5-3

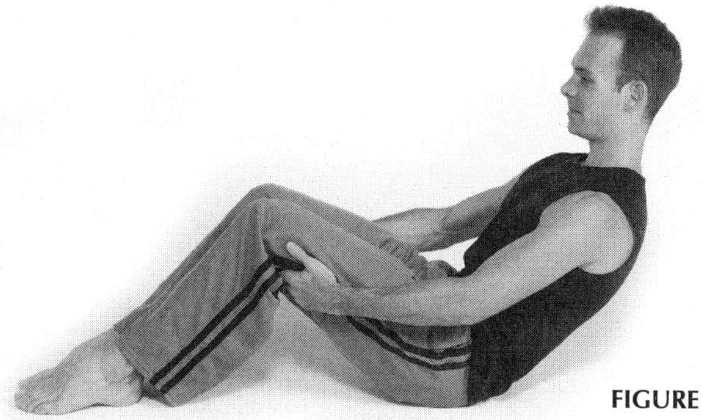

FIGURE 5-4

Start The Foundation Exercise
Step One **(FIGURE 5-4)**

1. Inhale fully.

2. Lengthen your exhale as you contract your abdominals, moving backwards into a deep C-curve. Aim the back of your waistline toward the floor. Look into your midsection.

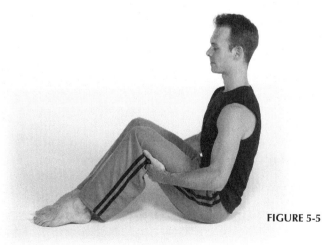

FIGURE 5-5

THE VISUAL IMAGERY GUIDE

Jᴀᴡ Cʟᴏsɪɴɢ

1. This abdominal contraction feels like your *ribcage and pubic bone forcefully draw together*. Visualize a *jaw clamping shut* within your trunk Exhale strongly, while practicing the power of the **closing jaw**.

2. Inhale as you tighten your abdominals while returning to sitting. **(FIGURE 5-5)**

THE FOUNDATION EXERCISE

For Step One: *Picture The Abdominal Muscles*

Muscle: *Rectus Abdominis*

THE VISUAL IMAGERY GUIDE

Fᴏʀ ᴛʜᴇ Dɪʀᴇᴄᴛɪᴏɴ ᴏꜰ ʏᴏᴜʀ Aʙᴅᴏᴍɪɴᴀʟ Cᴏɴᴛʀᴀᴄᴛɪᴏɴ: A Jᴀᴡ Cʟᴏsɪɴɢ

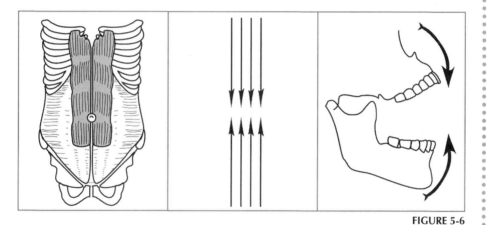

FIGURE 5-6

| **RECTUS ABDOMINIS** | **DIRECTION OF MUSCLE FIBERS AND CONTRACTION** | **IMAGE FOR ABDOMINAL CONTRACTION: JAW CLOSING** |

This is the outermost layer of your abdominals.
THE MUSCLE FIBERS RUN VERTICALLY.
They originate at the pubic bone and insert beneath the breastbone.

Keep your abdominals tight while you *Continue With Step Two ...*

Step two:

Exhale powerfully as you contract your abdominals moving backwards again into your C-curve. **(FIGURE 5-7)**

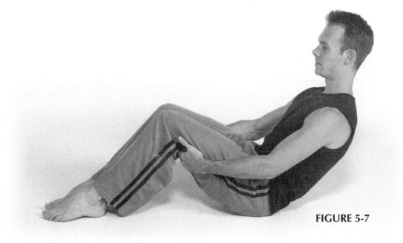

FIGURE 5-7

THE VISUAL IMAGERY GUIDE

UPPER CORSET

This abdominal contraction feels like tying the strings of a corset. Picture these strings attached to the bottom of each one of your ribs in the *front of your body*. Exhale powerfully, while feeling the *corset strings forcefully pulled together, inward, and downward along the front of your body toward your hips.* Begin by cinching your **corset** around your ribcage and then move it into your pelvis.

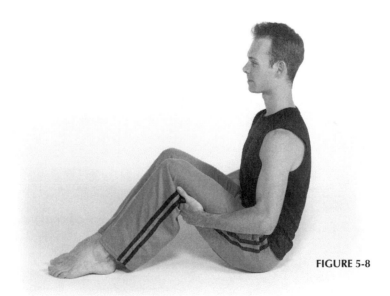

FIGURE 5-8

Inhale, *keeping* the abdominals contracted while returning to sitting. **(FIGURE 5-8)**

For Step Two:

Picture The Abdominal Muscles

Muscle: *External Obliques*

THE VISUAL IMAGERY GUIDE

Upper Corset

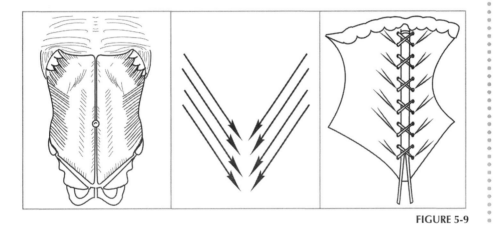

FIGURE 5-9

| EXTERNAL OBLIQUES | DIRECTION OF MUSCLE FIBERS AND CONTRACTION | IMAGE FOR ABDOMINAL CONTRACTION: CORSET |

This is the second layer of your abdominals.
THE MUSCLE FIBERS RUN IN DIAGONAL SLANTS.
They originate at the lower eight ribs and insert at the top of the pelvis.

Keep your abdominals contracted while you *Continue With Step Three ...*

For Step Three:

Exhale forcefully as you contract your abdominals, moving backwards into your C-curve. (FIGURE 5-10)

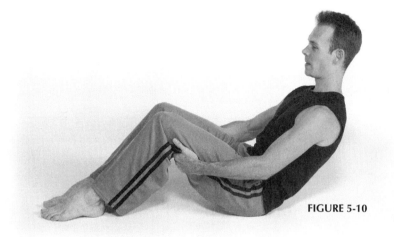

FIGURE 5-10

THE VISUAL IMAGERY GUIDE

LOWER GIRDLE

1. Exhale, while feeling the powerful elastic action of a **lower girdle** drawing your abdominal wall *in, back, and up*. The center of your body takes on a hollow scooped-out bowl shape. This is what Pilates refers to as your "scoop". The scoop starts by drawing the abdominals upward away from your pubic bone, in toward your spine, and finally up underneath your ribcage.

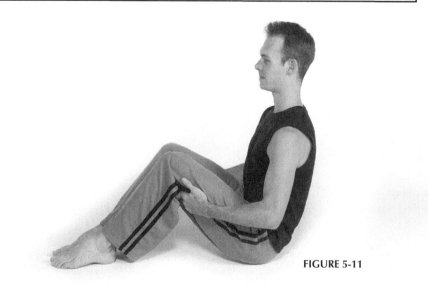

FIGURE 5-11

2. Inhale as you *keep* your abdominals engaged while returning to sitting. (FIGURE 5-11)

For Step Three:

Picture The Abdominal Muscles

Muscle: *Internal Obliques*

THE VISUAL IMAGERY GUIDE

Lower Girdle

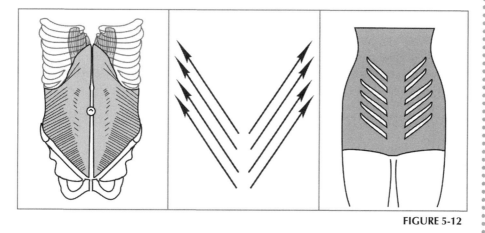

FIGURE 5-12

| INTERNAL OBLIQUES | DIRECTION OF MUSCLE FIBERS AND CONTRACTION | IMAGE FOR ABDOMINAL CONTRACTION: GIRDLE |

This is the third layer of the abdominals.
The MUSCLE FIBERS RUN IN DIAGONAL SLANTS.
They originate at the pelvic rim and insert on the last four ribs.

Keep your abdominals tight while you *Continue With Step Four ...*

For Step Four:

Exhale strongly as you activate your abdominals, moving backwards into your C-curve. **(FIGURE 5-13)**

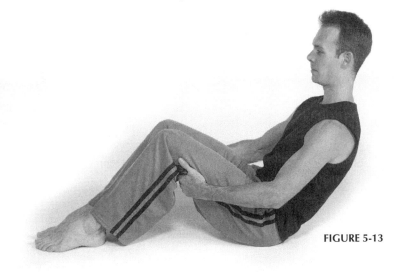

FIGURE 5-13

THE VISUAL IMAGERY GUIDE

HUG

1. This abdominal contraction feels like a low seat belt being drawn together across your stomach. While exhaling, visualize your abdominal muscle fibers powerfully *sliding and interweaving across each other like an internal* **hug**.

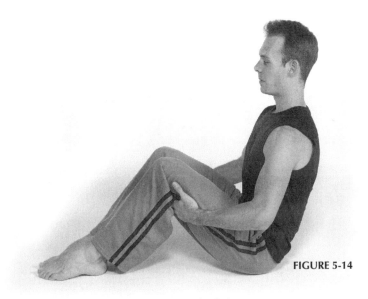

FIGURE 5-14

2. Inhale keeping the abdominals engaged while returning to sitting. **(FIGURE 5-14)**

THE FOUNDATION EXERCISE (CONTINUED)

For Step Four:

Picture The Abdominal Muscles

Muscle: *Transversus Abdominis*

THE VISUAL IMAGERY GUIDE

Internal Hug

SUCCESS

IN EVERY PILATES MOVEMENT YOU FIRST "FIRE" THIS DEEPEST LAYER OF YOUR ABDOMINALS. Cough to feel them.

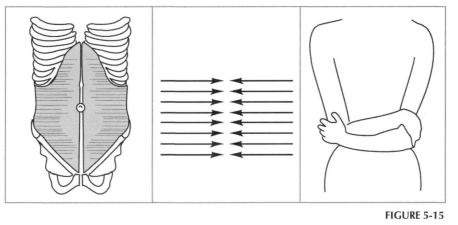

FIGURE 5-15

| TRANSVERSE ABDOMINIS | DIRECTION OF MUSCLE FIBERS AND CONTRACTION | IMAGE FOR ABDOMINAL CONTRACTION: HUG |

This is the fourth and deepest layer of your abdominals.
THE MUSCLE FIBERS RUN HORIZONTALLY.
They originate at the pelvic rim and the cartilages of the last six ribs. They insert at the breastbone and pubic bone.

Keep your abdominals tight while you *Continue With Step Five ...*

For Step Five:

Exhale as you contract your abdominals, moving backwards into your C-curve. **(FIGURE 5-16)**

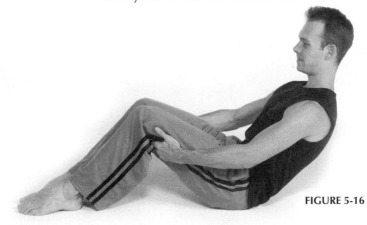

FIGURE 5-16

THE VISUAL IMAGERY GUIDE

NAVEL TO SPINE

1. Picture your upper trunk as a shirt to feel this abdominal contraction. While lengthening the sound of your exhale, imagine firmly tucking this shirt into your pants, then fasten the belt of your pants tightly together at your waistline, feel the closing of your belt sink your **navel inward toward your spine.**

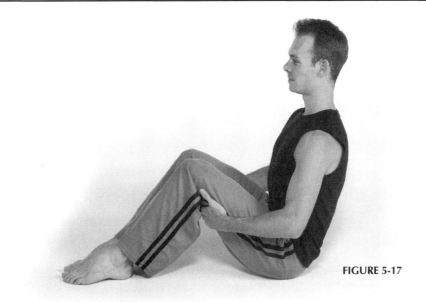

FIGURE 5-17

2. Inhale returning to sitting. **(FIGURE 5-17)**

Finish

Do not relax your abdominal muscles between the five steps of **The Foundation Exercise**! The visual imagery helps you inwardly shape and continuously contract the layers of your abdominals. After completing these five steps, your abdominals feel like they have gone through to your backbone.

For a Healthy Back:

THE FOUNDATION EXERCISE (CONTINUED)

For Step Five:

PICTURE THE MUSCLES BEHIND YOUR ABDOMINAL WALL

Muscles: *Iliopsoas and Multifidus*

THE VISUAL IMAGERY GUIDE

Navel to Spine

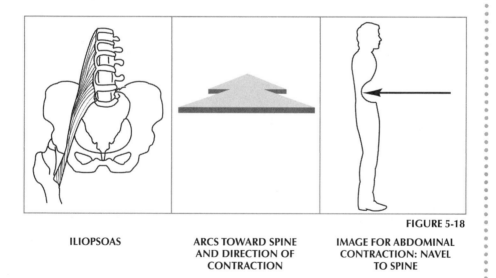

FIGURE 5-18

| ILIOPSOAS | ARCS TOWARD SPINE AND DIRECTION OF CONTRACTION | IMAGE FOR ABDOMINAL CONTRACTION: NAVEL TO SPINE |

The *iliopsoas* is the collective name for two muscles: the *psoas major* and the *iliacus*, but they are often called "*the psoas.*"

The hip flexors or *psoas* provide a *structural bridge* between the trunk and legs. It has two functions—spine flexion and hip flexion.

The *iliopsoas* and *multifidus* lie beneath the abdominal wall. They are near your spine. THEY WORK WITH THE ABDOMINALS TO *ANCHOR* THE LOWER BACK.

The Foundation Exercise gives you better access to these important *body organizers.*

Practice *one layer* of **The Foundation Exercise** several times in a row—to really *feel* your abdominals contract. For example, contract your *rectus abdominus* while imagining the motion of a **jaw closing** along the front of your trunk…*inhale keeping the muscles tightened,* exhale to close the jaw together tighter…inhale, then exhale drawing your stomach muscles together even more. Do this anytime throughout the normal course of your day to tone up your stomach muscles. You do not have to curve your spine. This exercise can be practiced in any position.

Memorizing the five images of **The Foundation Exercise** will give you the *key* to finding the power of your center, and toned stomach muscles. Keep repeating to yourself, "**jaw closing, corset, girdle, hug, and navel to the spine**". *Perform the five steps of* **The Foundation Exercise** *again as you say,* "*jaw-corset-girdle-hug-navel*". Your abdominals can move and shape internally. **REMEMBER, each image defines the direction of the internal abdominal contraction …**

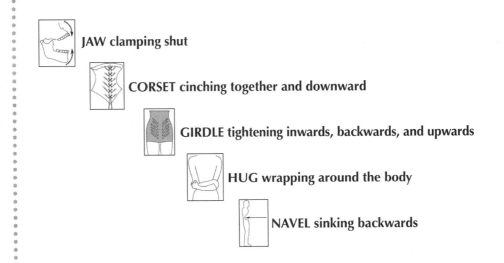

JAW clamping shut

CORSET cinching together and downward

GIRDLE tightening inwards, backwards, and upwards

HUG wrapping around the body

NAVEL sinking backwards

BREATHING REVIEW FOR THE FOUNDATION EXERCISE

Whether you are taking air in or letting it out the abdominals, NEVER RELAX. Maintain your abdominal contraction during your inhalations. Exhale forcefully to help contract the deep abdominal muscles.

The Foundation Exercise encourages breathing into the lower ribcage three-dimensionally. During your *inhales* focus on expanding the ribcage laterally. Allow the breath to open the back of the ribcage. *Exhale* through pursed lips, elongating the breath sound. This breath pattern encourages the engagement of the *transversus abdominis*. The **Foundation Exercise** helps develop an awareness of your deeper stabilizing muscles. In all mat exercises the breath and awareness of stabilization should occur *before* the actual movement.

SUCCESS

*Use **The Foundation Exercise** and **Three-Dimensional Breathing** for your Mat Program*

1. The inhalation in Pilates should not just emphasize the lateral direction. The use of the **Three-Dimensional Breathing** during Pilates exercises will help you breathe along the entire back surfaces of your body—the shoulder blade area, middle, and lower back. It includes directing air under your breastbone and into your armpits.

2. *There will be less expansion to the front of the body during the inhalation while performing Pilates movements. This is because the abdominal contraction is always maintained during the inhalation and exhalation of every Pilates movement!*

3. On each inhale, your diaphragm contracts and lowers. On each powerful exhalation, you squeeze your deepest abdominal layer—the *transversus abdominis*. It attaches all around the lower border of your ribcage, and connects with your diaphragm. The diaphragm can rise back up to its original dome shape as air leaves the lungs.

4. Your breathing energizes your body so you can find your abdominal muscles Concentrate on deeply contracting your abdominal muscles, while breathing powerfully. This is the key to every Pilates movement.

SUCCESS

Use **Three-Dimensional Breathing** and **The Foundation Exercise** during your Desk Freedom and mat exercises. They help you to continuously contract your abdominals during repetitions of each exercise, as well as throughout the breathing cycle.

SUCCESS — CHALLENGE

*Reverse **The Foundation Exercise***

Visualize…the four abdominal muscle groups from the deepest layer to the outermost layer.

      1. Navel to the spine
        2. Hug
          3. Girdle
            4. Corset
              5. Jaw Closing

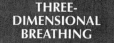

FOUNDATION EXERCISE

See Page 83

THREE-DIMENSIONAL BREATHING

See Page 74

HOW IT HELPS

- **The Foundation Exercise** provides an internal massage for the organs, which lie behind your abdominal wall. It can improve digestion, circulation, and elevate your energy level. This may help to boost the immune system. Exercise increases the inner core body temperature. This can enhance the body's resistance to colds and flu. A well-conditioned center promotes an active healthy life.

- **The Foundation Exercise** can be used anywhere, while in any position to routinely find the power of your core. Perform it lying down, sitting, standing, and walking. Do it with your muscles only. Your bones do not have to move. There is a subtle change in your posture. Note how this internal exercise makes you feel more alert and alive. No one around you knows that you are performing it. This practical internal exercise is for work, traveling, or anytime! It is an empowering technique to fight off stress of any kind. The exercise generates higher levels of energy; a necessity for our busy lives today. Moving from your core promotes ease and efficiency of motion. Your center integrates all of your movements.

- It makes everyday repetitive movements easier, more efficient, and graceful. Try an experiment when you get in and out of the car. Pay attention to your stomach muscles, and how you breathe. Most of us completely relax our stomach muscles, and either inhale, or hold our breath. Instead, powerfully exhale while pulling your abdominals inward toward your spine.

- A strong center decompresses your spine.

- **The Foundation Exercise** enhances proper breathing. You are able to fully expand and deflate your lungs. It is excellent for exercising your respiratory system.

- It provides stability and mobility for lifting heavy objects. It protects your joints and back. *Persistent practice of **The Foundation Exercise** becomes a "mental trigger," or reminder, to activate your center in order to conquer unexpected physical tasks with confidence.*

- *Creative visualization is an important part of any fitness, dance, sport, or Pilates session. **The Foundation Exercise** helps you to draw upon the mental image of centering to support each movement. You experience every repetition anew, and it is never boring. Use it for safety, success, and results. Activate your abdominals for every **Desk Freedom or mat exercise.***

- When skaters, gymnasts, or dancers have a bad day they complain that they cannot find their center. Athletes can practice their sports skills using **The Foundation Exercise** to achieve that extra edge, and soar past competitors. You stay centered for training sessions. This carries over to peak performance. Try it for bursts of energy, as well as for improving stamina, speed, and motor control.

- People who train with free weights and machines at the gym can benefit by using **The Foundation Exercise**. Implement it into every repetition of your workout. Use your abdominals hundreds of times in one fitness session. The result will be a strong, toned stomach. It provides safety for your back and joints. This centering technique energizes your workouts. Always move from your core in the gym.

- Use it in Yoga, T'ai Chi, and the martial arts. Center-oriented movements invigorate your body and mind. Yoga teaches that the center is the place where we connect to the energies of the universe. Centered movements develop your physical balance. This opens the door to trusting your gut instincts and intuition. From this place of relaxed alertness you feel physical, mental, emotional, and spiritual harmony.

Chapter Six
The Desk Freedom Exercises

The **Desk Freedom Exercises** make healthy use of your office time. This is a program of muscle-easing movements that can be done in your chair. They maximize your body's need for exercise, especially in an office environment. It takes only a few minutes. Fit them into your workday. Keep a copy of the exercises at your desk. Insert the movements into small break periods throughout the day. They relax your body as you hold the phone and align your posture at the computer. Some of the improvements are less eyestrain, better concentration, more stamina, and a positive outlook. These exercises, which deeply relax and energize you, give you a tangible sense of your daily stress slipping away.

We spend hours of our life at a desk. This program serves as motivation to keep changing your sitting positions. Good posture will help your back stay healthy. When you do stand up from your desk you are well aligned and free of knots. A few moments of focused movement time becomes an opportunity to be aware of your body's "internal environment." Office movements are primarily small, repetitive gesture-like movements. These full-range-of-motion exercises are a workout for your entire body.

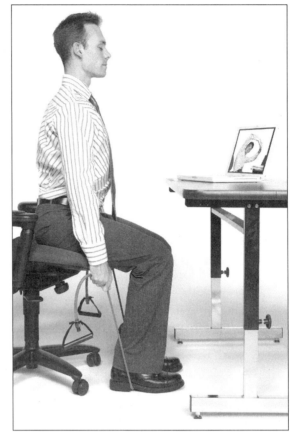

FIGURE 6-1

A Quick Pick-Me-Up
*Perform the **Sit Up and Take Notice Exercise** with a Prop* **(FIGURE 6-1)**

To Warm-Up for the Desk Freedom Exercises
Keep a tie, towel, or elastic exercise band at your desk.

1. Place it underneath the arches of your feet.

2. Hold onto each end of the prop.

3. "Walk" your hands down the prop until it is taut.

*Do this while you perform the following steps of **The Sit Up and Take Notice Exercise:***

1. Stack your hips, ribs, chest, and head on top of each other like building blocks.

2. Sit tall on top of your sit-bones. Your sit-bones are located at the base of your pelvis. Rock from side to side to feel these bones.

3. Press the soles of your feet into the floor as if they are growing roots into the earth. Feel this strong connection to the ground through your feet and legs.

4. Stretch your body up toward the ceiling away from your feet.

Keep contracting your inner thighs, buttocks, and deep abdominal muscles. Take slow, powerful breaths.

Breathing Tips for The Desk Freedom Exercises

Keep your breathing continuous, slow, and even throughout the exercises. Tone up your stomach, buttocks, and leg muscles by tightening them more with each exhalation. Try to make this a habit and the focus of your exercises. Concentrate on moving your abdominal region. Pull your abdominals in toward the spine. Initiate all of your movements from your abdominal area. You will be opening up a whole new world of physical movement.

THE DESK FREEDOM EXERCISES

Perform the following exercises daily while sitting at your desk, on an airplane, and watching TV. These exercises can also be done while standing.

SHOULDER AND SPINE FREEDOM EXERCISE

Prepare with Sit Up and Take Notice Exercise

1. Sit tall on top of your sit-bones. Your sit-bones are located at the base of your pelvis. Find these bones by rocking side to side.

2. Stack your hips, ribs, chest, and head on top of each other like building blocks.

3. Press the soles of your feet into the floor as if they are growing roots into the earth. Feel this strong connection to the ground through your feet and legs.

4. Stretch your body up toward the ceiling away from your feet.

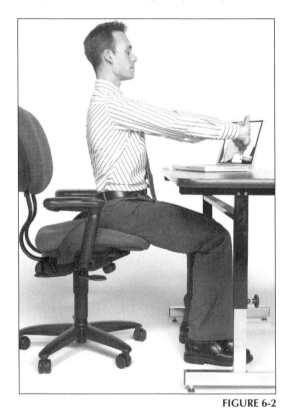

FIGURE 6-2

Start

Step One (FIGURE 6-2)

1. Clasp your hands together with your fingers intertwined. Turn your palms to face *away* from you.

2. Stretch your arms forward slightly below shoulder level.

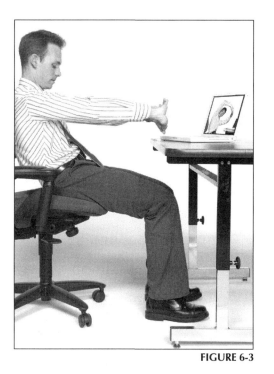

FIGURE 6-3

Step Two

3. Each time you exhale tighten your abdominals.

4. Contract your abdominals while rounding your spine into a C-curve shape.
FIGURE 6-3

THE VISUAL IMAGERY GUIDE

Step Three

- Imagine you can put your NAVEL ONTO YOUR SPINE with each exhale.
  Think of continuously tightening your abdominal muscles in, back, and up.

Finish

Uncurl the spine.

Repeat several times.

SUCCESS

Navel to spine is often referred to as the Pilates "scoop." It is the physical motion of drawing your abdominal muscles *inward* and *upward*. Especially the *tranverse* abdominals: these are the deepest layer of muscles near your spine. The result is a hollow or scooped out appearance in the waistline.

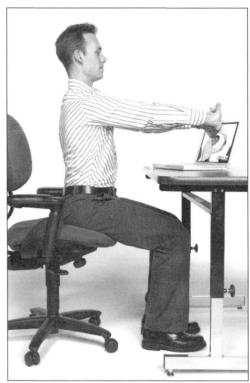

FIGURE 6-4

SAFETY
Omit this exercise if you have had a recent back injury.

SIT UP AND TAKE NOTICE

See Page 43

Prepare with The Sit Up and Take Notice Exercise

Start

Step One (FIGURE 6-4)

1. Clasp your hands together with the fingers intertwined.

2. Turn your palms to face *away* from you.

3. Stretch your arms forward slightly below shoulder level.

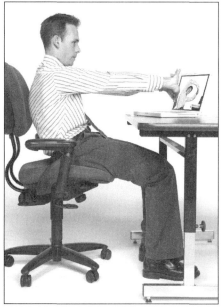

FIGURE 6-5

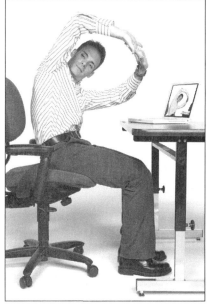

FIGURE 6-6

Step Two (FIGURE 6-5)

1. Round your body into a deep C-curve.

2. On your exhales, sink your navel deeper and deeper toward your spine.

Step Three (FIGURE 6-6)

1. Stay in your C-curve.

2. Bend your elbows.

3. Dip the *left elbow toward the floor*.

4. The *right elbow points up toward the ceiling*.

5. Look through your arms. Notice that your arms frame your face.

6. Your upper trunk is twisted toward the right. You are looking to the right.

THE VISUAL IMAGERY GUIDE

Step Four

Imagine that during your exhales you can CLOSE THE FRONT OF YOUR RIBCAGE TOGETHER—LIKE A CORSET. FEEL YOUR ENTIRE SHOULDER GIRDLE DROP DOWNWARD INTO YOUR WAISTLINE. THIS IS LIKE TUCKING YOUR SHIRT INTO YOUR TROUSERS.

Change sides.

Repeat several times.

ENERGIZED BREATHING, CHEST, SHOULDER, AND NECK FREEDOM EXERCISE

SAFETY

Omit this exercise if you have had thoracic surgery. If you have shoulder problems reach back only within a pain-free range.

SIT UP AND TAKE NOTICE

See Page 43

Prepare with Sit Up and Take Notice Exercise

Start

Step One (FIGURE 6-7)

1. Sit forward on the edge of your chair.

2. Place your hands behind your body on the back of the chair.

Step Two

1. Squeeze your shoulder blades together.

Step Three

1. On your inhales, breathe into the back of your rib cage.

2. On each exhale, powerfully contract the abdominal muscles in, deeper toward your spine. Open the chest, but don't allow your ribs to pop out. Close the front of your ribcage together—like a corset.

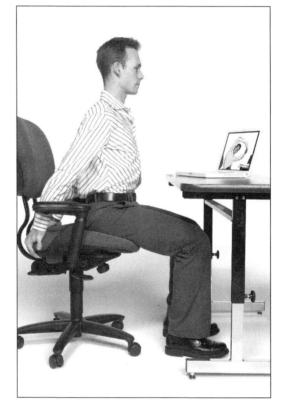

FIGURE 6-7

THE VISUAL IMAGERY GUIDE

Step Four

FEEL YOUR SHOULDER BLADES SLIDE DOWN AWAY FROM YOUR NECK AND HEAD. PICTURE THEM GLIDING INTO THE BACK HIP POCKETS OF YOUR TROUSERS.

Repeat several times.

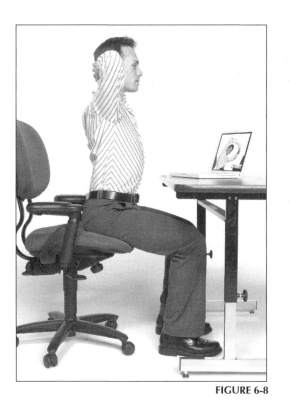

FIGURE 6-8

SAFETY

If you have a weak neck do the stretch without using your arms.

Prepare with Sit Up and Take Notice Exercise

Start

Step One (FIGURE 6-8)

1. Layer your hands and place them behind the head. The fingers are not intertwined.

2. Keep your elbows wide. Stabilize your shoulder blades. Imagine gently pulling them down the back.

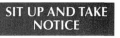

SIT UP AND TAKE NOTICE

See Page 43

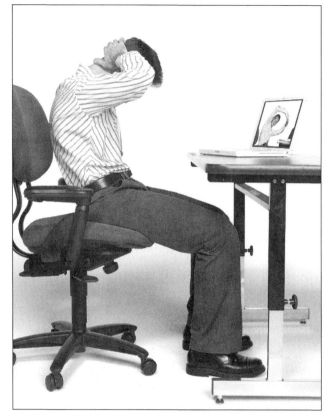

FIGURE 6-9

Step Two (FIGURE 6-9)

1. Lower your head a few inches.

2. Rest your hands gently on your head, without pulling.

3. The chin is not scrunched to your chest. Instead, you have curved your upper body forward. Imagine an orange between your chin and chest.

THE VISUAL IMAGERY GUIDE

Step Three

PICTURE A GIANT BALLOON LOCATED IN BETWEEN YOUR SHOULDER BLADES. INHALE. VISUALIZE THE BALLOON EXPANDING. EXHALE AND THE BALLOON DEFLATES. *Take several full breaths*. They are long, slow, even, and tranquil inhalations and exhalations. Sink your navel deeper toward your spine while exhaling.

Slowly return upright.

Repeat several times.

STOMACH, SPINE ARTICULATION, AND BACK FREEDOM EXERCISE

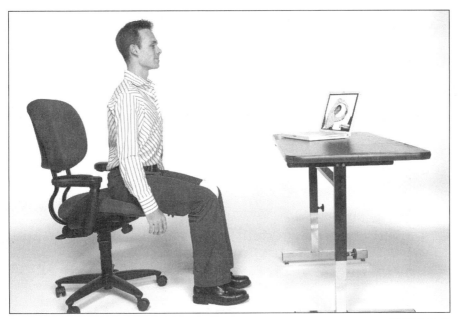

FIGURE 6-10

Prepare with Sit Up and Take Notice Exercise

Start

Step One (FIGURE 6-10)

1. Sit on the edge of your chair.

2. Press your legs together tightly.

3. Contract your buttock muscles.

4. You can place an **Amazing Sock Ball**, or even this book in between your knees. This helps you activate the proper leg, buttock, and abdominal muscles. Squeeze the legs and buttocks towards the prop.

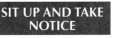

SIT UP AND TAKE NOTICE

See Page 43

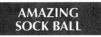

AMAZING SOCK BALL

See Page 117

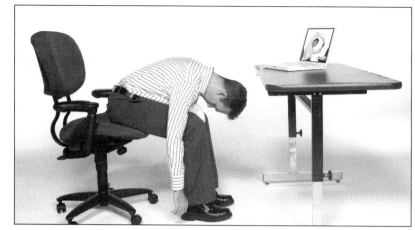

FIGURE 6-11

Step Two (FIGURE 6-11)

1. Exhale while powerfully contracting your abdominal muscles.

2. Curl your torso toward the floor, flexing at your hips.

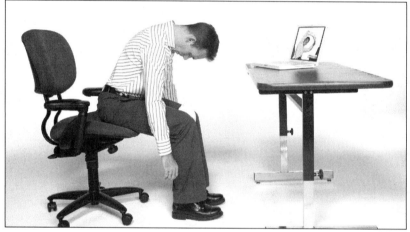

FIGURE 6-12

Step Three (FIGURE 6-12)

3. Press the soles of your feet into the floor.

4. Squeeze your inner thighs and buttock muscles together again.

5. Keep tightening your abdominal muscles, legs, and buttocks while uncurling the spine.

THE VISUAL IMAGERY GUIDE

Step Four

IMAGINE THERE IS A WALL BEHIND YOU. ROLL THE SPINE DOWN AND ROLL THE SPINE UP. Visualize the wall behind you while you un-stack and stack your spine. Move one vertebra at a time while you roll down and up.

Repeat several times.

Easy Breathing, Waistline, and Trunk Rotation Freedom Exercise

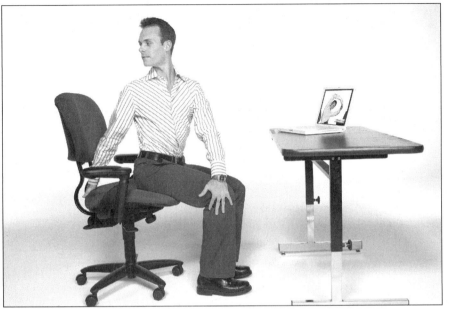

FIGURE 6-13

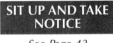

SAFETY

Omit this exercise if you have a rib or back injury. If you have a shoulder problem, reach back only within a pain-free range.

Prepare with Sit Up and Take Notice Exercise

Start

Step One (FIGURE 6-13)

1. Sit at the edge of your chair. Inhale filling the back of your ribcage. Exhale tightening your abdominals.

2. Twist your body to the right. Initiate this spinal rotation from your lowest ribs. Keep your hipbones facing forward.

3. Gaze over your right shoulder.

Step Two

1. Keep the abdominals scooped inward toward your spine.

2. Breathe deeply into your upper trunk.

Your inhalations expand your ribcage sideways. Use the power of your exhalations to strongly contract your abdominal muscles. Your abdominal muscles physically push the air out of your lungs. Joseph Pilates called this "wringing out your lungs."

SIT UP AND TAKE NOTICE

See Page 43

111

Change to the other side.

Repeat several times.

SPINE, BUTTOCKS, OUTER THIGH, AND LOWER BACK FREEDOM EXERCISE

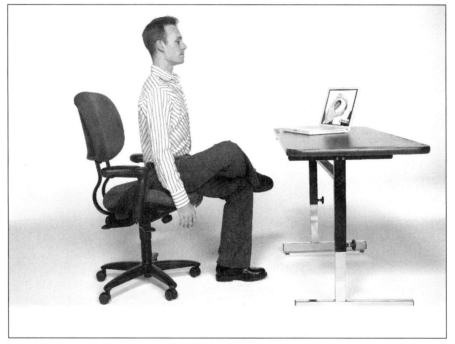

FIGURE 6-14

Prepare with Sit Up and Take Notice Exercise

SIT UP AND TAKE NOTICE

See Page 43

Start

Step One (FIGURE 6-14)

1. Sit on the edge of your chair.

2. Cross your right ankle over your left knee.

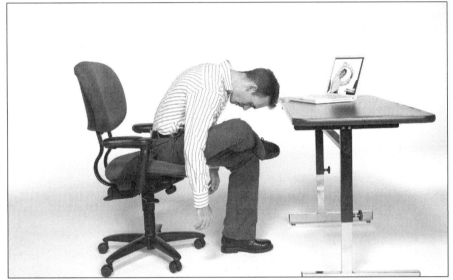

FIGURE 6-15

Step Two (FIGURE 6-15)

1. Curl your torso toward the floor.

2. Initiate this movement by tightening your abdominals. Powerfully contract them *inward and upward* toward the tops of your ears.

THE VISUAL IMAGERY GUIDE

Step Three

IMAGINE YOU ARE ROLLING FORWARD AND OVER A HUGE WAVE.
Your trunk traces the longest possible arc in space. Uncurl the spine.

Change sides.

Repeat several times.

SIT UP AND TAKE NOTICE

See Page 43

FOUNDATION EXERCISE

See Page 83

THREE-DIMENSIONAL BREATHING

See Page 74

AMAZING SOCK BALL

See Page 117

FOOT FAN

See Page 124

ROOTS

See Page 126

SUCCESS

Use Your ABCs For Each of **The Desk Freedom Exercises**

- Prepare with **Sit Up and Take Notice** for each exercise. Add **The Foundation Exercise**, and **Three-Dimensional Breathing**, to connect the mind to the body for more results.

- Warm up with **The Foundation Exercise** and **Three-Dimensional Breathing.** You will be using internal exercises. Everyone around you is unaware that you are getting an energy boost. **The Foundation Exercise** strengthens your abdominal muscles and massages the lungs and internal organs. **Three-Dimensional Breathing** is a bath for the lungs. It both energizes your body and calms your mind. It is a valuable stress management tool for a fast-paced work life.

When you incorporate any of these ABC exercises into **The Desk Freedom** movements—you are integrating centering into your workouts. Centering involves your alignment, breathing, and core abdominal muscles. You can make important physical changes to your body and improve your health right at your desk.

Use an **Amazing Sock Ball**, or even this book to tone your inner thighs, pelvic floor, buttocks, and abdominal muscles. Place it in between your thighs, above your knees during most of the stretches. Squeeze the prop using your inner thigh and buttock muscles. This helps you access more abdominal muscles and lengthens your body. You will trim your tummy and tighten your inner thighs and buttocks.

Take your shoes off and give your feet a break with **Foot Fan** and **Roots**. Keep an **Amazing Sock Ball** at your desk for a soothing back and hip massage. Place it behind your body. Sit against the back of your chair. Press your back muscles into the Sock Ball. Keep moving the ball to a different spot. Breathe deeply. Use the ball on the muscles not the spine.

Chapter Seven
The Amazing Sock Ball

Treat yourself to an Amazing Sock Ball massage daily. It is amazing how deeply relaxed your body will feel. The Sock Ball is an invaluable healing tool for many aches and discomforts. It is not always easy to get to the source of tension. The massage movements combined with the weight of your body on the ball lengthen muscle fibers. Just one session can alleviate tension and increase circulation. It improves the flow of blood and oxygen to the body. Self-massage is not included in most Pilates' programs, yet it relieves tight muscles and chronic tension. Speed up your results by using the Sock Ball to warm-up or cool-down.

HOW TO MAKE A SOCK BALL

Use three pairs of athletic socks.

Step One
Twist the toe of a sock into a small *tight* ball.

Step Two
Turn the remainder of the sock inside out over the ball you have made.

Step Three

Repeat these first two steps until you are out of sock.

Step Four

Slide this ball into the toe of the next sock.

Step Five

Repeat steps one through four until you have a Sock Ball twice the size of a tennis ball.

Experiment with the size until it is just right for you. It is an oval-shaped ball. The ball is approximately six inches by four inches. You may have to re-make it from time to time. It will get a lot of use.

THE BENEFITS OF A SOCK BALL

The oval shape allows you to mold your body onto the ball. For a *deeper massage*, place the egg-shaped ball vertically on a spot. For a *lighter massage*, place the ball horizontally.

- The larger you make your Sock Ball, the greater the increase in pressure.
- It releases more points at once.
- It molds to your body for deeper relaxation.
- The Sock Ball provides the ability to vary the angle in which it presses into a muscle.
- Moving the ball by a ¼ of an inch makes a big difference. The knots of muscular tension dissolve.

THE AMAZING SOCK BALL MASSAGE

Perform while lying down, sitting, waking, going to sleep, watching TV, at the computer, on an airplane, at your hotel, etc. Use it during warm-up or cool-down for athletics/dance/recreational/performance activities, and between fitness workouts, or any endeavor to relieve muscle soreness and fatigue.

SAFETY

Use the Sock Ball only on the muscles. Keep it away from the bones and spine.

Preparation for The Amazing Sock Ball Massage

Lie down on a firm surface. Use a mat or blanket. You may prefer a small pillow under your head. Make sure you are comfortable.

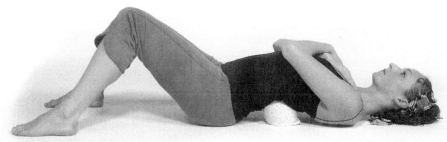

FIGURE 7-1

Start the Sock Ball Massage (FIGURE 7-1)

• Lie on your back. Place the Sock Ball beneath one of the following areas: upper, middle, or lower back, hips, or scalp.

• Lie on your stomach. Place the Sock Ball beneath one of the following areas: forehead, cheek, chest, or stomach.

• Lie on your side. Place the Sock Ball beneath one of the following areas: cheek, trunk, hips, or legs.

Step One

1. Make sliding movements. Soften your body against the ball. *Keep reminding yourself to take long, slow, tranquil breaths.* This will enhance the relaxation of your muscles.

2. Try small movements of your body in many directions: forward and backward, to the right side and to the left side, and circling. Breathe.

Step Two

1. Use the weight of your body against the ball. Let go and dissolve into the ball.

2. Keep moving it to a different spot. Breathe.

3. Slowly roll on it. Breathe.

THE VISUAL IMAGERY GUIDE

FOR YOUR SOCK BALL MASSAGE

Step Three

- Breathe deeply. Imagine your intake of air has a color. See it spread and soothe each area you are massaging.

- Remain still on one spot. Visualize melting your body into the ball.

- Imagine the ball as the healing hands of a masseuse. You can get a full body massage.

This massage gently peels away the layers of tightness that accumulate within the muscles. The increased oxygen and blood flow improves your youthful complexion.

Greet the world with an open expression. Trust your own intuition for what feels best during your Sock Ball massage.

DON'T LEAVE HOME WITHOUT YOUR AMAZING SOCK BALL!

When traveling by plane, etc., place the Sock Ball behind your back against your seat. Move it to different spots along your hips, back, and head. Take long, slow, even, tranquil breaths. It will relieve minor aches and pains so you arrive at your destination stress-free.

HOW IT HELPS

We think we have to live with many of our body's aches and pains. The first time you use **The Sock Ball**, you will say it is "amazing." Just try it!

- It is helpful for anything from headaches to sore muscles.

- It relieves joint and muscular discomfort and tightness.

- It alleviates muscle spasms and helps re-establish lost range of motion. This is important in athletics, fitness, and rehabilitation. If you are stuck in bed it is a useful healing tool.

- It can soothe sinus problems and tightness in the jaw.

- It improves circulation to the upper body and therefore the complexion.

- It relaxes tight muscles so you can get a good night's sleep.

- Use it along your stomach area to improve digestion.

- It helps alignment, flexibility, organ function, and stress relief.

Chapter Eight
The Athletic Foot

Our automobile tires provide balance and support for our car. Our feet do the same for our body. Yet we put more time into maintenance for our car tires than we do our feet. Our feet must take us to our many destinations in life. We take our feet for granted most of the time. Only when we have a problem with them do we realize how restricted we are.

A regular foot massage can melt away the tension we carry within our feet. This results in an open, malleable, and grounded foot. The feet can then do the job of efficiently transmitting movement up through the legs and into the rest of the body. Often the idealized foot is small and delicate. Yet wide, supple, and strong feet can act as shock absorbers and propel the body into motion. Healthy feet provide a solid, stable base of support.

These exercises make your feet feel alive and grounded. **The Five-Minute Foot Massage, Foot Fan, and Roots** will help you regain the feet you were born with. Your arches lift, your ankles strengthen, and your toes move independently of one another.

FOOT REFLEXOLOGY

Foot reflexology is one of the oldest forms of massage. It teaches that every point on the foot relates to specific organs or muscles in the body. These are "energy centers." Reflexology maintains that a foot massage not only soothes tired, achy feet, but also promotes a feeling of well being throughout the entire body. A foot massage improves circulation. It increases the flow of blood and oxygen to the whole body. Think of it this way: every body of water has sediment at the bottom that builds up. Even our feet could use a good internal cleansing to rid them of unwanted debris.

THE FIVE-MINUTE FOOT MASSAGE

Perform while sitting, watching TV, at bedtime, and traveling. It is also an excellent addition to your yoga/dance/sports/mat workouts. Use it for warm-up or cool-down.

You can even give yourself a routine foot massage when you are watching television.

- Apply plenty of pressure like kneading dough.

- It should feel great—a "good hurt."

- At first you will be surprised at the tender or sore spots. Soreness usually does not mean you should avoid that area. Continue to work on that spot so the discomfort dissipates.

- It is more relaxing when you breathe deeply during your foot massage.

Three Locations for your Five-Minute Foot Massage

Location One (FIGURE 8-1)
The Bottom of the Foot

- Apply pressure with your thumbs along the bottoms of the feet, pressing, squeezing, and kneading from the heels up to the toes. Work up and down your foot along the main arch. Use the weight of your body to lean into the massage motion from your hands.

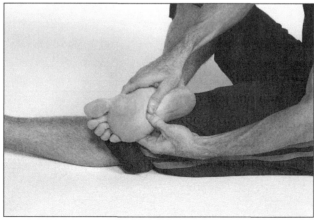

FIGURE 8-1

121

Location Two

Where the Ankle Meets the Foot

- Use both of your hands. Massage in a full circle around your ankle.

- Work the area called the "ankle foot"—where the ankle meets the foot. *It is located in the front of the lower leg.* (**FIGURE 8-2**)

- Press into the area called the "heel foot"—where the ankle meets the heel of the foot. *It is located in the back of the lower leg.* This is a pinch-like or grabbing motion. Use your entire hand and thumbs. (**FIGURE 8-3**)

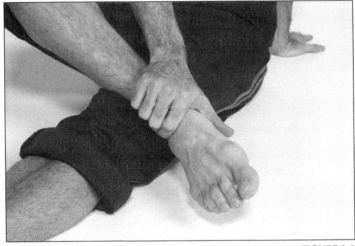

FIGURE 8-2

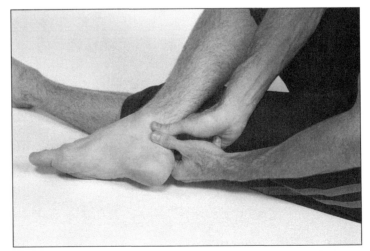

FIGURE 8-3

Location Three

The Top of the Foot (FIGURE 8-4)

- Massage the fleshy areas between the bones. These areas are like the webbings of a duck's feet.

- Start in between the toes.

- Follow this *groove* back and forth from your toes toward your ankle. There are a total of *four* of these grooves.

- Press deeply into these valley-like areas. There is a lot of tension stored there.

Finish by grabbing the foot with both hands. Put your thumbs on the sole and fingers on the top. Wring it out as if squeezing water out of a towel.

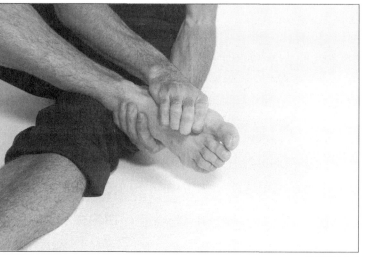

FIGURE 8-4

HOW IT HELPS

- Be creative with your routine **Five-Minute Foot Massage**. It will relieve stress and feel great.

- You will be more sure-footed and confident.

- The massage and the following exercises relieve foot problems.

- They will enhance your movement and balance skills for this fitness program, sports, dance, and everyday life. We are reducing tension in the entire body when our feet are massaged.

THE FOOT FAN EXERCISE

Perform while sitting or standing, on an airplane,
traveling, or anywhere.

THE VISUAL IMAGERY GUIDE

Have you ever watched a cat stretch its paw apart to clean in between its toes?

Start The Foot Fan Exercise

• From a sitting position, place only your heels on the ground. Lift the rest of your feet. Spread your toes apart as far as you can like your feet are taking a huge "yawn."

Visualize this stretch not only coming from your toes but from your entire foot and ankle. **(FIGURE 8-5)**

• Keep your feet spread open like a fan.

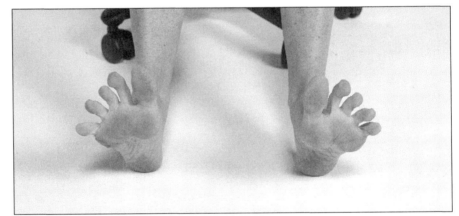

FIGURE 8-5

- Next flatten each toe into the floor *one by one.* **(FIGURE 8-6)**

- Begin with your little toe and work consecutively to your big toe.

- Still keep your feet and toes stretched open, as wide as possible, while placing them onto the floor.

Do this several times.

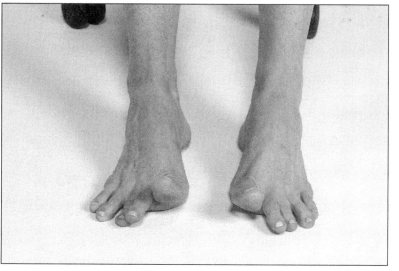

FIGURE 8-6

THE ROOTS EXERCISE

Perform while sitting or standing, on an airplane,
traveling, or anywhere.

Start The Roots Exercise while sitting
During this exercise keep the heels and toes on the floor.

1. Draw the toes backwards toward the heels. **(FIGURE 8-7)**

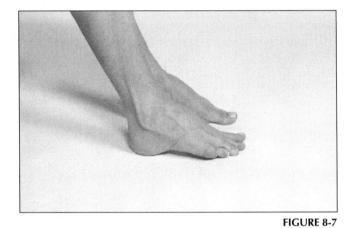

FIGURE 8-7

• Your *arches* will rise further away from the floor. The feeling is like the suction of a vacuum cleaner hose getting stuck on one spot on a carpet.

• The outer and inner sides of your feet move equally.

• *Keep the toes flat. Check to see that the knuckles of your toes do not rise up away from the floor. Imagine roots growing out of your toes. They spread out and sink deep into the earth.*

Repeat this several times.

If your feet cramp during this exercise, repeat the **Five-Minute Foot Massage**. It is evident that your feet require some routine attention.

Also try combining the **Foot Fan Exercise** and **Roots Exercise** for more dexterity and strength. *Move directly from* **Foot Fan** *into* **Roots** *several times!*

THE ROOTS EXERCISE WITH A SOCK PROP

*You can perform **Roots** by placing a loose sock under your toes. Grab onto the sock with your toes.*

THE ROOTS EXERCISE WITH A MIRROR

*It is interesting to do **Roots** standing in front of a mirror. Watch what happens to your ankles.*

- Check your foot, ankle, and leg alignment *before* you begin. Do your ankles cave inward or outward? **(FIGURE 8-8)**

- During **Roots** observe your ankles adjusting into a central position. Your ankles align with your lower leg and feet. **(FIGURE 8-9)**

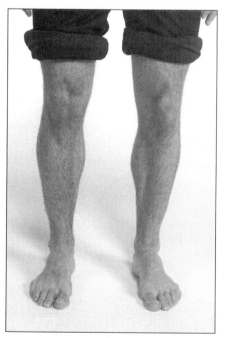

FIGURE 8-8

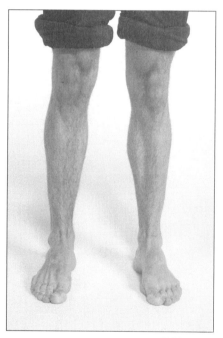

FIGURE 8-9

THE ROOTS EXERCISE IN REVERSE

Try reversing The Roots Exercise.

- Keep the heels and toes on the floor.

- The feet remain in the same place on the floor.

- Draw the heels forward toward the toes.

The size of your arch will increase, to varying degrees.

HOW IT HELPS

HOW THE **FIVE-MINUTE FOOT MASSAGE**, THE **FOOT FAN**, AND THE **ROOTS EXERCISE** HELP YOU

In personal habits, care for the feet comes last, if at all. Healthy feet are open, supple, and powerful. These exercises provide better balance, grace, and alignment for anything you do. They reinforce proper sequencing from the feet into the hips and continuing up along the spine. Keep foot and balance problems at bay and de-stress your feet by using these exercises.

These exercises help you to feel grounded during any activity. They will improve your overall performance in the mat program. When your feet are in contact with the mat, you recruit the proper muscles.

Part Two

*Your At-Home Stretching Program,
Basic Pilates Mat Program, and
Sports Mat Program*

Chapter Nine

Stretching is the Key to Youth

A supple body is an ageless body. Stretching keeps you feeling youthful. A routine stretching program is an important fitness component for a healthy adult. It helps your muscles and connective tissue stay elongated and elastic. This improves circulation.

Tense muscles contribute to stress. Supple muscles create deep relaxation. Stretching keeps your muscles from shortening and enhances the range of motion in your joints. It improves your posture and balance. Lack of flexibility in the muscles and joints puts extra stress on them. It can cause inflammation and overuse syndromes. The risk of injury increases considerably when muscles become short and tight. Stretching also improves concentration, digestion, and sleep patterns.

You can stretch daily. Children move and stretch their bodies into different positions all day. Watch a cat or dog after they take a nap. They stretch themselves before they begin walking.

Stretching is non-competitive. It is not important how far you go in a stretch but rather how it feels while you're in a stretch.

**THREE-
DIMENSIONAL
BREATHING**

See Page 74

Preparation for your Stretching Program

• Find a space large enough for your body to stretch out fully in all directions.

• You will need a cushioned mat or blanket, or you can place a towel on a carpet. An extra towel can serve as a pillow. Elevate your head slightly for more comfort.

• This time is just for you. Work out away from outside distractions. Some light music may enhance your relaxation.

• Assist your stretches by using a small towel or strap. This is helpful if you have tight hamstrings, which are located along the back of your thighs.

• The *support leg* is the leg that holds the body's weight or stabilizes the body.

• The *gesture leg* is the leg that does not support the body's weight.

• Remember to use your ABCs during each stretch.

    A. Maintain a neutral spine.
    B. Use your **Three-Dimensional Breathing**.
    C. On every exhalation, gently sink your navel to your spine.

SAFETY

• A *static* stretch is a stretch that you *hold*. This allows the "stretch reflex" to kick in. This means that when you stay in a stretch position the muscles relax a bit more. Hold each stretch for a minimum of thirty seconds, and as long as a minute.

• Stretch to the point of "comfortable tension," never pain. In any movement, if it feels bad, it is. Stretching too far may cause soreness.

• Move slowly and smoothly into and out of your stretches.

• Try to relax your entire body during a stretch.

• Stretch after a fitness or sports activity. The muscles are "warm." When a muscle is "cold" you can tear muscle fibers. You may decide to stretch before an activity, but first warm up with a five-minute walk.

SUPINE: HAMSTRING STRETCH

Muscles: Hamstrings and Hips

Position:

- Lie flat on your back on the floor.

- Your **left support leg** is bent. The sole of the foot is on the floor.

- Raise your **right gesture leg**. Point your knee toward the ceiling. It is now at *center* in a *parallel* position.

- Use your hands at the back of the gesture leg to move your thigh toward your chest.

Start
Use your ABCs.

Step One (FIGURE 9-1)
- Slowly extend your right leg. Keep it slightly bent to avoid straining your hamstrings.

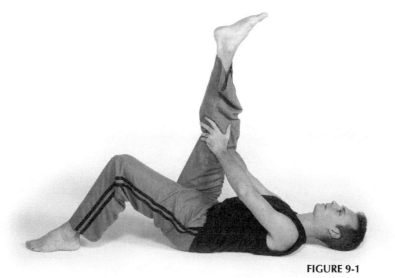

FIGURE 9-1

- Keep your bottom on the floor. Check that your spine is in "neutral." The back and neck are lengthened.

- Flex your foot to add a calf stretch.

- Gently lower the leg to come out of the stretch.

Now repeat the stretch with the other leg

**THE PRINCIPLES
OF MOVEMENT –
ABCs**
*Alignment • Breathing
Centering and Core Stability*

Variation of your Supine: Hamstring Stretch (FIGURE 9-2)

• Use a towel or strap instead of your hands to hold onto your leg. It may be helpful for the above stretch and for the following exercises.

• Wrap the strap around the back of the straight gesture leg. Hold both ends of the strap.

• Draw the right leg toward your chest.

• Relax the upper body.

You may also want to place the strap around the bottom of your foot. This adds a stretch down the entire back of the leg.

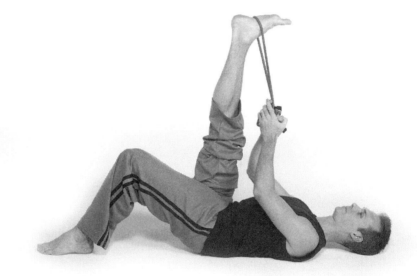

FIGURE 9-2

SUPINE: HAMSTRING AND INNER THIGH STRETCH

Muscles: Hamstrings, Adductors, and External Rotators

Position:

• Lie flat on your back.

• Your **left support leg** is bent. The sole of the foot is on the floor.

• Raise you **right gesture leg**.

• Use your hands at the back of the right gesture leg to move it out to the *side* of your body. It is now in an *externally rotated position.*

Start
Use your ABCs.

Step One (FIGURE 9-3)
• Slowly extend your right leg. Keep it slightly bent.

• Keep your bottom on the floor. Check that your spine is in "neutral." The back and neck are lengthened.

• Flex your foot to add a calf stretch.

Now repeat the stretch with the other leg.

**THE PRINCIPLES
OF MOVEMENT –
ABCs**

*Alignment • Breathing
Centering and Core Stability*

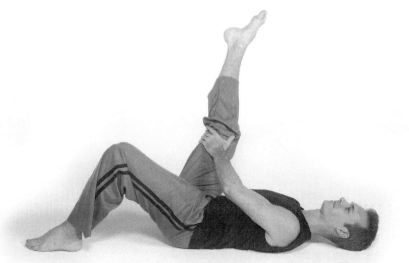

FIGURE 9-3

SUPINE: HAMSTRING AND OUTER THIGH STRETCH

Muscles: Hamstrings, Abductors, and Internal Rotators

SAFETY

Omit this exercise if you have had a hip replacement.

Position:

- Lie flat on your back.

- Your **left support leg** is bent. The sole of the foot is on the floor.

- Raise your **right gesture leg**.

- Use your hands at the back of your gesture leg to move your thigh *across* your body toward your left side. It is now in an *internally rotated* position.

Start
Use your ABCs.

Step One (FIGURE 9-4)
- Slowly extend your right leg. Keep it slightly bent.

- Hug your leg toward your body.

- Check that the spine is in "neutral". The back and neck are lengthened.

- Flex your foot to add a calf stretch.

Now repeat the stretch with the other leg.

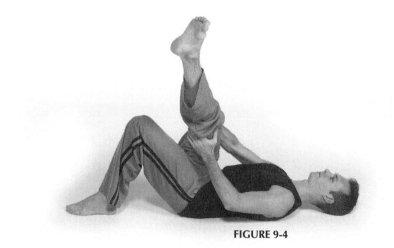

FIGURE 9-4

Variation for your Supine: Hamstring Stretches

• In the three previous stretches keep the gesture leg in its designated position (center, to the side of your body, or across your body).

• Then, externally rotate it one inch.

• Next, internally rotate it one inch.

The additional stretches of your leg in external and internal rotation improve the range of motion in your hip joint. The hamstrings relax more. It is also helpful for back care. Your lower back and buttock muscles gently stretch and relax.

SUPINE: BUTTOCKS AND LOWER BACK STRETCH

Muscles: Buttocks and Lower Back

SAFETY

Omit this exercise if you have had a hip replacement.

Position: (FIGURE 9-5)

• Lie on your back. Feet are flat on the floor.

• Raise your right leg.

• Place your right ankle across your left knee.

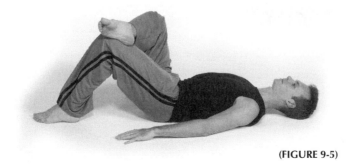

(FIGURE 9-5)

Start
Use your ABCs.

Step One (FIGURE 9-6)

• Bring both legs off of the floor.

• Hold on behind the left leg with your hands.

• Draw both legs toward your chest.

• Keep the pelvis on the floor. Check that your spine is in "neutral." The back and neck are lengthened.

Repeat the stretch with the other leg.

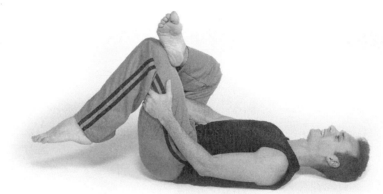

(FIGURE 9-6)

SUPINE: TRUNK ROTATION STRETCH

Muscles: Torso and Hips

SAFETY

Omit this exercise if you have had a recent back injury.

Position: (FIGURE 9-7)

• Lie down on your back.

• Both legs are bent.

• The feet are flat on the floor.

• Your arms are extended out to your sides at shoulder level.

• Palms on the floor.

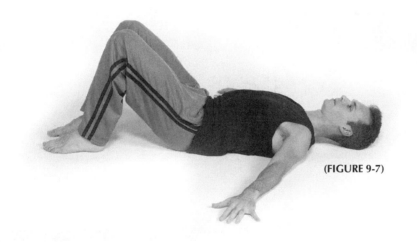

(FIGURE 9-7)

Start
Use your ABCs.

Step One (FIGURE 9-8)

• Rotate your hips *as one unit* to your left.

• The head stays center.

• Eyes look up to the ceiling.

**THE PRINCIPLES
OF MOVEMENT –
ABCs**

*Alignment • Breathing
Centering and Core Stability*

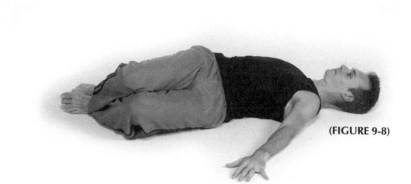

(FIGURE 9-8)

Step Two

• Tighten your abdominals *before* you return to your back. Return the hips as a unit.

Change sides.

FITNESS LEVELS

INTERMEDIATE
ADVANCED

Variation of the Supine: Trunk Rotation Stretch

Step One (FIGURE 9-9)

• Lie down on your back.

• Both of your legs are extended.

• Lift your right leg off of the floor. Bend it at a 90-degree angle. This will be your **gesture leg**.

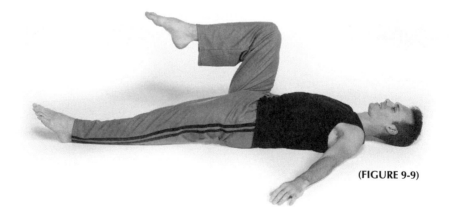

(FIGURE 9-9)

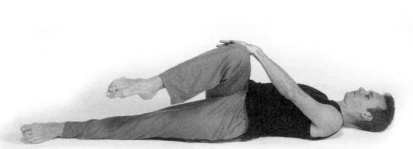

(FIGURE 9-10)

Step Two (FIGURE 9-10)

- Place your left hand on your right knee.

- Exhale. Tighten your abdominals. Rotate your hips as one unit to your left.

- Stretch your right arm out to the side. Relax the shoulders toward the floor. Head stays center.

- Eyes look up at the ceiling.

Step Three

- Tighten your abdominal muscles *before* you return to your back. This stabilizes your lower back. Return the hips as a unit.

Change sides.

LYING ON YOUR SIDE: THIGH STRETCH

Muscles: Quadriceps and Hip Flexors

SAFETY

Omit this exercise if you have a knee problem.

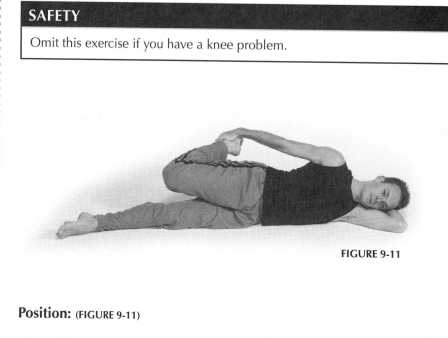

FIGURE 9-11

Position: (FIGURE 9-11)

- Lie on your left side with your right leg bent at 90 degrees.

- Place your left arm under your head. Prop your head up with a towel as a pillow for extra comfort.

- Use your right hand to hold onto your right lower leg or ankle.

Start
Use your ABCs.

Step One
- Draw your right heel toward your bottom.

- Your right upper leg is in line with your hips and spine.

- Your spine is in "neutral." The back and neck are lengthened. Tighten your abdominal muscles to stabilize your lower back.

Change sides.

ABDOMINAL STRETCH

Muscles: Abdominals, Chest, Arms, and Upper Back

SAFETY

Omit this exercise if you have had a recent back injury or if you have any vertebral abnormalities.

If you experience any shoulder or wrist strain, slide the arms further forward.

Position: (FIGURE 9-12)

• Lie on your stomach.

• The palms of your hands are flat on the floor directly under your shoulders.

• Your elbows are bent and close by your sides.

• The legs are straight and slightly apart.

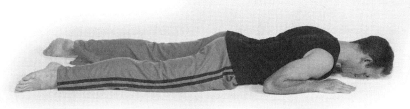

(FIGURE 9-12)

Start
Use your ABCs.

Step One (FIGURE 9-13)
• Slowly raise your upper body off of the floor. This posture is called the Cobra in yoga.

• Lengthen up through the chest.

• You are supported on your forearms.

• *Look down at the floor.* Keep the back of your neck long.

• Lower your shoulders away from your ears.

143

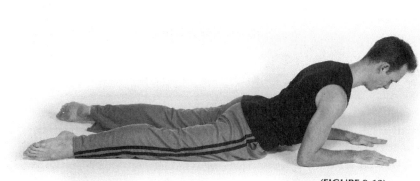

(FIGURE 9-13)

Step Two

• Tighten your abdominal and buttock muscles.

• Extend your legs away from your hips.

• Keep the length in your spine. Maintain the lower back in "neutral".

• Lower your body to rest.

Repeat 3-5 times.

SAFETY

Reverse this stretch afterwards by rounding your back. Finish in the fetal position while lying on your side.

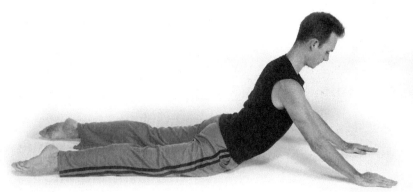

(FIGURE 9-14)

Variation of the Abdominal Stretch

Step One (FIGURE 9-14)

• Move your palms further apart and *forward* of your shoulders.

• Exhale. Contract your abdominals.

• Lengthen up through your chest.

• Straighten your arms but keep the elbows soft.

Step Two

• Maintain the length through your spine.

• Reach your legs outward from your hips, pressed against the mat.

• Your neck is long. *Your eyes look down slightly.*

• The shoulder blades are gently pulled back and down.

• Inhale as you return to the ground.

Repeat 3- 5 times.

Finish

End by curling your back into the fetal position while lying on your side.

THE VISUAL IMAGERY GUIDE

VISUAL IMAGERY GUIDE FOR YOUR STRETCHING PROGRAM
Visualize the following while holding a stretch:

• Picture a flowing river running through your muscles.

• Let the force of gravity work for your body. Melt your body further and further into the earth. Feel the weight of your body.

• Allow the muscles of the entire body to become as relaxed as possible while holding a stretch. Become an "inner detective". Take a survey of each body part, one at a time. Breathe, and take a moment to consciously relax your feet, ankles, etc., until you reach your head. This technique is called "progressive relaxation." It is an excellent technique for stress reduction. Use it during your stretches. Also, try it alone for deep relaxation while lying down on your back.

• Add oppositional lengthening to your stretch program. Feel your body softly lengthen in two different directions at once while you hold a stretch.

HOW IT HELPS

In our society even the simplest movements have become rushed and constricted. Your **Stretching Program** is executed slowly. It is a de-stressor. Individual variants in flexibility depend upon genetics, daily movement habits, posture, emotional stress, and participation in movement activities.

Stretching involves deep relaxation breathing and concentration. The key to improving flexibility is to focus on your breathing. During each stretch use the **Three-Dimensional Breathing** exercise. Conscious awareness of your breathing during a stretch creates more lasting benefits. Focus on your breathing if your mind wanders. Breathing is the vehicle for relaxing the muscles and calming your mind.

Stretching benefits anyone involved in vigorous physical activity. Proper flexibility training enhances sports performance and alleviates sore muscles. It prevents injury because there is less tissue resistance. It speeds up recuperation time after physical exertion.

Stretching can relieve low back pain. It pinpoints tight muscles and joints. Stretching enhances the body's blood and nutrient supply. Tense muscles have more toxicity and can cause lethargy. Stretching gives us a sense of vitality. It increases the quantity of synovial fluid within our joints, which keeps them healthy. Stretching calms the nerves. It improves neuromuscular coordination.

Energize your stretching program. Use **The Foundation Exercise**. This adds core control. Use these stretches before or during your mat exercises.

THREE-DIMENSIONAL BREATHING

See Page 74

FOUNDATION EXERCISE

See Page 83

Chapter Ten

Basic Pilates Mat Program

TEACHING TIPS

*For the **Basic Pilates** and **Sports Mat Programs***

The following tips will help you to evaluate and master your mat exercises.

- The essence of Pilates is the attention to details.

- Many principles are involved in one simple movement. Focus on the imagery to bring *all* of the principles together. Your body will then move as an efficient unit.

- Keep your mind on your muscles to see results: a longer, leaner, and more toned body.

- Becoming your own coach is how your body will change. Cultivate your "inner detective" to check each aspect of a movement. Your practice of Pilates will then inspire you for a lifetime.

Use your ABCs, Alignment, Breathing, and Centering exercises. Practice the helpful visual imagery guides from Chapters Three, Four, and Five for every one of the mat exercises.

PELVIS AS A FISH BOWL

See Page 56

FOUNDATION EXERCISE

See Page 83

THE COMPASS

See Page 52

THREE-DIMENSIONAL BREATHING

See Page 74

OPPOSITIONAL LENGTHENING

See Page 45

TEACHING TIPS

The following is a checklist for *each* exercise:

Alignment and Centering

☐ Are you beginning each exercise in "neutral"? Use *The Pelvis as a Fish Bowl Exercise* to find "neutral."

☐ Are you keeping your shoulders relaxed and your neck long? Slide your shoulder girdle toward your feet. Lift your pelvic floor and abdominal muscles in the opposite direction of the shoulder girdle, up, up, up, toward the top of your head.

☐ Are you using *The Foundation Exercise* to fully engage all four layers of your abdominal muscles? Focus on *The Foundation Exercise* to feel your deepest layer of abdominals, the transverses abdominals. For example, imagine your ribcage is a corset that can cinch together. Also visualize drawing the corset strings downwards toward your hips. Sink your navel to your spine. Use your Powerhouse to *prepare for and execute every exercise.*

☐ Is the base of your Powerhouse engaged? Activate the base of your Powerhouse. Squeeze your buttocks and inner thighs together and lift your pelvic floor muscles upward.

☐ Use *The Compass* imagery to ground your feet into the mat during the exercises.

Breathing and Centering

☐ Is your breathing slow and powerful? Use your *Three-Dimensional Breathing* to "stoke your engine" and find your deep abdominal contractions.

☐ Become a graceful athlete by "dancing" *each* movement. Be precise and blend one movement fluidly into the next. Lengthen your inhales and exhales to create this elegant exercise rhythm.

☐ Was the movement challenging? It should be. Are you using oppositional lengthening?

Preparation for your Basic Pilates Mat Program

- Use a firm cushioned mat.

- You may prefer to use your **Amazing Sock Ball** to help you activate the base of your Powerhouse. Place the Sock Ball between your thighs, above your knees. Squeeze your buttock muscles. *Visualize your outer thighs pressing your inner thighs together.*

TEACHING TIPS

REPETITIONS OF AN EXERCISE
Perform between three to ten repetitions of an exercise.

- The emphasis is never on the number of repetitions.

- Focus on the quality and *slow* rhythm of the movements.

- Pay attention to your body's limits.

- You may need to relax and stretch in between the exercises. If you do, lie on your back and bring your legs in towards your chest.

The Visual Imagery Guides in this chapter will help you focus on your technique. Concentrate on the images while performing the exercises to access all of your **principles of movement** and your Powerhouse. Paint a vivid picture in your mind of the images. Remember the imagery exercises in Part 1 were designed for you to practice throughout your day. *They help reinforce the important principles of movement to attain more results from your mat workouts. For example, stand in the middle of your compass, zipper your leg and buttock muscles together, slide your shoulder blades into your back trouser pockets,* and do the **Three-Dimensional Breathing and Foundation Exercise** all at once! Focus your complete attention on the visual images anytime, anywhere, and often. Utilizing your mind-body connection daily is the key to success in the mat program. *The imagery helps you prepare, initiate, and execute each movement. Stabilize first—then move. Slide your shoulder girdle downward, navel back, front ribs in and down, buttocks squeezed, upper thighs glued together and breathe deeply. This all happens at once!*

THE HUNDRED

*This exercise is called **The Hundred** because of the breathing rhythm. The breathing pattern warms up your Powerhouse for the exercises to follow. Take long, slow inhales and exhales. Try not to pant.*

SAFETY

Avoid lifting your head if you have neck problems.

THE VISUAL IMAGERY GUIDE

Centering

Whether you are breathing in or out, continuously contract your abdominals. Use *one* of the following images to activate your abdominal muscles:

- **Jaw closing-corset-girdle-hug-navel to the spine.** Experiment with the images to find one that helps you feel your abdominals, and stabilize your back.

- **Picture pumping springs into the mat with the entire length of your arms.**

- Organize your shoulder girdle using the following images:
    1. **Slide your shoulder blades into your back trouser pockets.**
    2. **Slide your arms pits into your side trouser pockets.**
    3. **Slide your collarbone into your waistband.**

This imagery will help you keep your shoulders relaxed and away from your ears. When you organize your shoulder girdle, it is easier to feel your abdominals contract inward toward your spine.

TEACHING TIPS

- You may need to begin performing this exercise with your head on the mat until your strength improves.

- You can support your head with one hand.

- Rest your head back onto the mat if you feel any neck discomfort and continue the exercise.

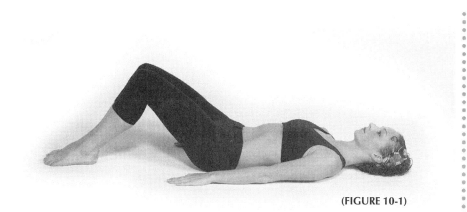

(FIGURE 10-1)

Preparation for The Hundred (FIGURE 10-1)

• Lie on your back.

• Your legs are bent with the feet flat on the mat. Place the heels approximately 2½ feet forward of your hips.

• Your legs are squeezed together so you can use the strength of your thighs and buttock muscles.

• Lengthen your arms by your sides with the palms facing down towards the mat.

• "Glue" your back to the mat by drawing your navel into your spine.

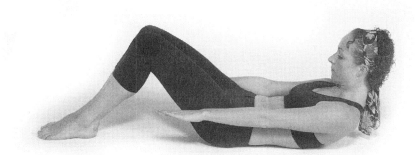

(FIGURE 10-2)

Start The Hundred (FIGURE 10-2)

• Bring your head toward your chest. Look toward your navel.

• Lift your shoulder blades off of the mat to engage your abdominals.

• Stretch your arms to the wall in front of you.

• **Breathe in** *for 5 counts as you pump your arms quickly up and down 5 times.*

151

• **Breathe out** for 5 counts as you pump your arms 5 times. This is **1 set.**

Perform **2-3 sets** at the beginning of this program.

Your eventual goal is to build this to **10 sets**, to equal a cycle of one hundred.

Finish

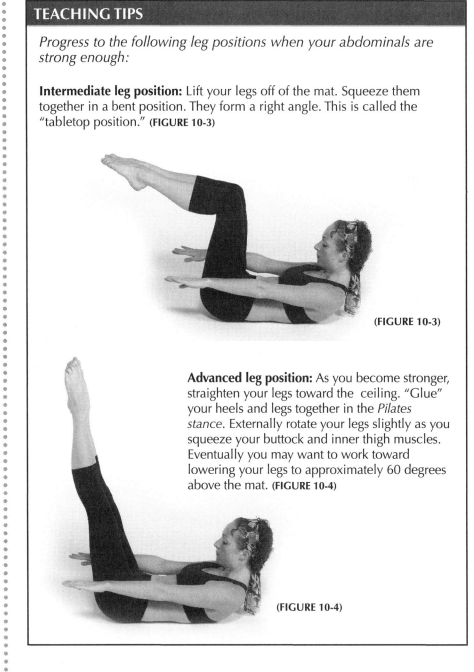

TEACHING TIPS

Progress to the following leg positions when your abdominals are strong enough:

Intermediate leg position: Lift your legs off of the mat. Squeeze them together in a bent position. They form a right angle. This is called the "tabletop position." **(FIGURE 10-3)**

(FIGURE 10-3)

Advanced leg position: As you become stronger, straighten your legs toward the ceiling. "Glue" your heels and legs together in the *Pilates stance*. Externally rotate your legs slightly as you squeeze your buttock and inner thigh muscles. Eventually you may want to work toward lowering your legs to approximately 60 degrees above the mat. **(FIGURE 10-4)**

(FIGURE 10-4)

Hug your knees to your chest. Prepare for the **Roll-Up.**

THE ROLL-UP

*This exercise will strengthen your abdominals in order
to control the movement articulation of your spine. Your back
and hamstrings will gain flexibility.*

SAFETY

Avoid this exercise if you have back or disc problems.

THE VISUAL IMAGERY GUIDE

Alignment

- Feel your feet sink into the mat. **Make your feet as malleable and open
  as a cat's paw. Visualize your feet on the middle of a compass. Ground
  and stretch your feet out to the north, south, east, and west directions
  of your compass.**

- **Picture your shoulder girdle area as a shirt that you tuck into the
  waistline of your pants.** Slide your shoulder girdle toward your feet as
  you roll up and down.

- **Imagine there are several tennis balls in between your legs—from your
  ankles to your knees and inner thighs. Squeeze your buttock and leg
  muscles firmly together against the tennis balls.**

- **Picture your body continuously curling over a huge wave while rolling
  up and down.** Use the power of your breathing to access your deepest
  abdominals.

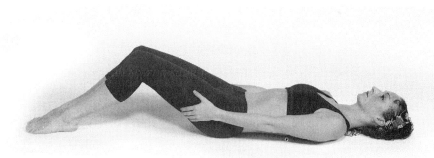

(FIGURE 10-5)

Preparation for the Roll-Up (FIGURE 10-5)

• Lie on your back.

• The legs are bent.

• Your feet are flat on the mat and approximately 2 ½ feet from your hips. When your feet are too close to your hips it is difficult to roll up and down with control.

• Hold onto the back of your thighs with your hands.

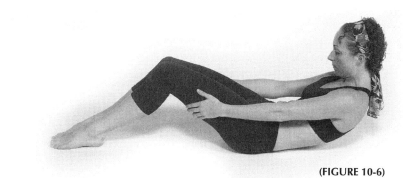

(FIGURE 10-6)

Start the Roll-Up
Step One (FIGURE 10-6)

• Inhale.

• Exhale, bringing your chin toward your chest. Imagine an orange between your chin and chest.

• Roll up to sitting one vertebra at a time.

• Walk your hands along the back of your legs toward your feet while curling up to sitting. This helps your spine form the letter **C** as you roll up and forward. Discontinue this when your abdominals become strong enough to control the **Roll-Up.**

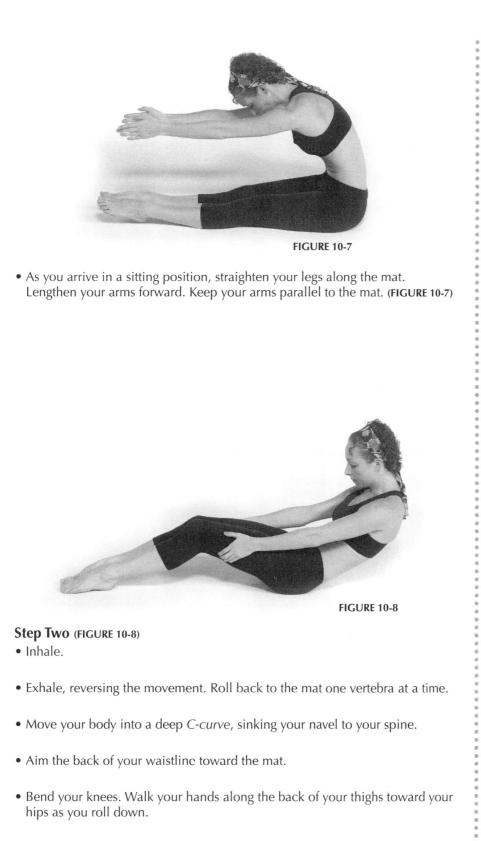

FIGURE 10-7

- As you arrive in a sitting position, straighten your legs along the mat. Lengthen your arms forward. Keep your arms parallel to the mat. **(FIGURE 10-7)**

FIGURE 10-8

Step Two **(FIGURE 10-8)**
- Inhale.

- Exhale, reversing the movement. Roll back to the mat one vertebra at a time.

- Move your body into a deep *C-curve*, sinking your navel to your spine.

- Aim the back of your waistline toward the mat.

- Bend your knees. Walk your hands along the back of your thighs toward your hips as you roll down.

Repeat 3-5 times.

1. When your abdominals are strong enough, begin the exercise by stretching your arms over your head. **(FIGURE 10-9)**

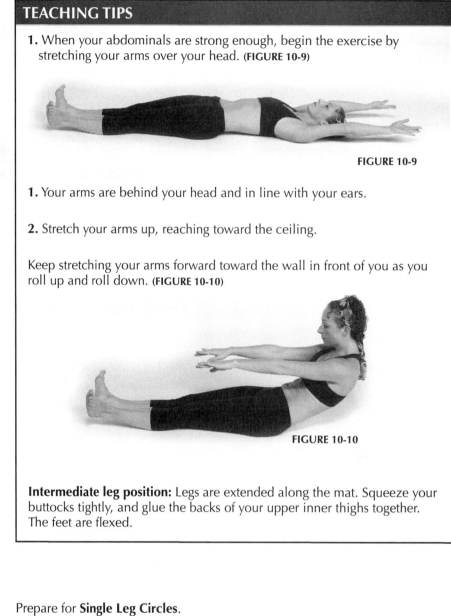

FIGURE 10-9

1. Your arms are behind your head and in line with your ears.

2. Stretch your arms up, reaching toward the ceiling.

Keep stretching your arms forward toward the wall in front of you as you roll up and roll down. **(FIGURE 10-10)**

FIGURE 10-10

Intermediate leg position: Legs are extended along the mat. Squeeze your buttocks tightly, and glue the backs of your upper inner thighs together. The feet are flexed.

Prepare for **Single Leg Circles**.

SINGLE LEG CIRCLES

This exercise strengthens your Powerhouse, hips, and legs.

THE VISUAL IMAGERY GUIDE

Alignment

- **Picture your circling leg as a paintbrush. Your foot is the brush.** Keep your foot long and relaxed as it paints circles in space.

- **Imagine your pelvis is a fish bowl. The rim of the bowl is your waistline.** Contract your deep abdominals and squeeze your buttock muscles to keep your hips still on the mat. There is no water sloshing out of your pelvic fish bowl.

TEACHING TIPS

- Make your leg circles small until your abdominals are strong enough to keep both sides of your hips anchored to the mat.

- Increase the size of your leg circles when your Powerhouse is strong enough to allow for flexibility in your hips.

- Feel the fluidity of the circular motion especially on the upward swing of the leg.

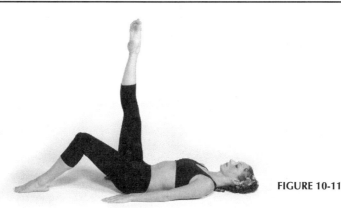

FIGURE 10-11

Preparation for Single Leg Circles (FIGURE 10-11)

- Lie on your back.

- Your left leg is bent.

- Your right leg is in a central position with your foot aimed toward the ceiling. It is straight and slightly turned out from the hip joint. You still get the benefits of this exercise with a slightly bent leg.

- Your arms are straight and by your sides on the mat.

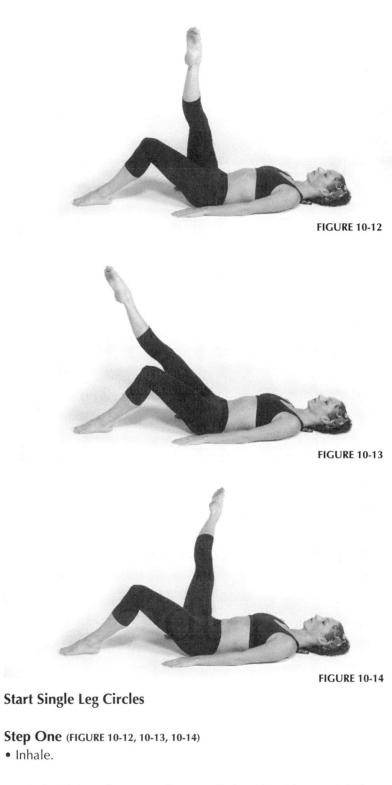

FIGURE 10-12

FIGURE 10-13

FIGURE 10-14

Start Single Leg Circles

Step One (FIGURE 10-12, 10-13, 10-14)

• Inhale.

• Exhale while making a small, controlled circle with your right leg.

• Circle your right leg in toward your bent leg, down, around, and up.

Repeat 5 times.

• Reverse the circle. Take your right leg out, down and back up to your central position.

Repeat 5 times.

Change legs.

Hug your knees to your chest. Place your legs long on the mat. Roll up one vertebra at a time. Sit toward the front of your mat for **Rolling Like a Ball.**

Preparation for Rolling Like a Ball

ROLLING LIKE A BALL

This exercise teaches balance and control from your Powerhouse. It provides a gentle massage for the spine.

SAFETY

If you have severe scoliosis, you may omit this exercise. Avoid this exercise if you have back problems.

THE VISUAL IMAGERY GUIDE

Centering and Alignment

• **Sink your navel toward your spine**. This helps you maintain a C-curve shape.

• **Visualize tucking a shirt into trousers.** This improves shoulder girdle organization and abdominal support.

TEACHING TIPS

• Use the abdominals to initiate the roll back. Sink your navel towards the spine and roll forward. Avoid gaining momentum from the legs.

• Maintain the curves of the spine without over-flexing the neck. Look at your navel.

• Avoid upper body tension by stabilizing your shoulder blades. Glide them toward your hips.

• Roll back to the base of your shoulder blades.

Step One: Starting Position (FIGURE 10-15)
- Balance behind your sit-bones in a C-curve, with the feet off of the mat.

- Place your hands on your shins.

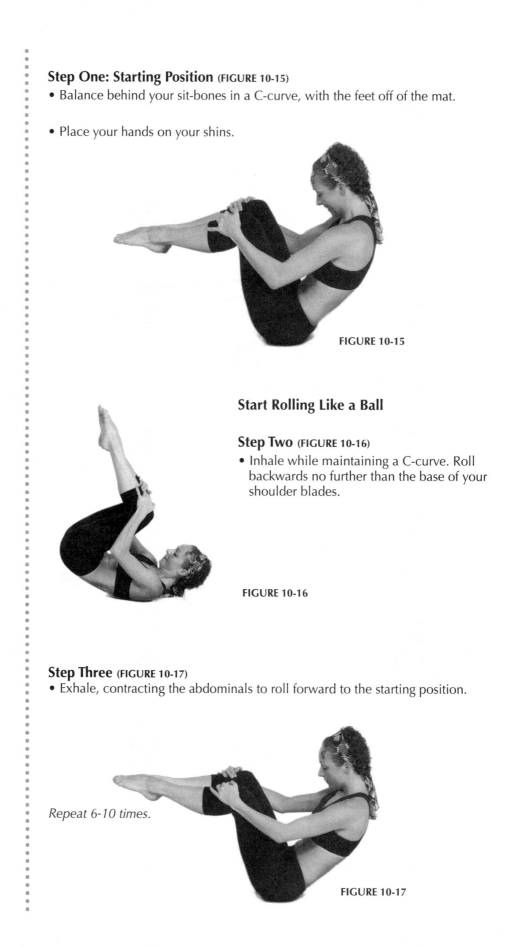

FIGURE 10-15

Start Rolling Like a Ball

Step Two (FIGURE 10-16)
- Inhale while maintaining a C-curve. Roll backwards no further than the base of your shoulder blades.

FIGURE 10-16

Step Three (FIGURE 10-17)
- Exhale, contracting the abdominals to roll forward to the starting position.

Repeat 6-10 times.

FIGURE 10-17

Place your hands by your hips. Move back to the center of the mat. Roll down one vertebra at a time to prepare for the **Single Leg Stretch**.

SINGLE LEG STRETCH

*This exercise strengthens your Powerhouse
and improves your alignment.*

SAFETY

If you have weak knees place your hands under your thighs. Keep your straight leg high until your abdominals are strong. Your back remains "glued" to the mat. Never lower your leg beyond your hips.

THE VISUAL IMAGERY GUIDE

Centering
- **Visualize your back sinking into wet cement.**

- Keep inwardly shaping your abdominals toward your spine. **Picture a heavy weight on your stomach carving and scooping your abdominals in, back, and up.**

TEACHING TIPS

- Coordinate your movements using your breathing.

- *Inhale for 2 changes of your legs and arms.*

- *Exhale for 2 changes of your legs and arms.*

- Keep your hip, knee, and foot in one long line.

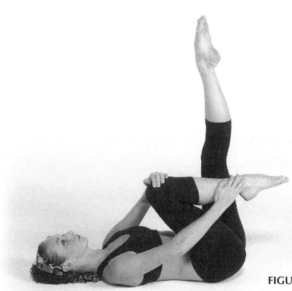

FIGURE 10-18

Preparation for Single Leg Stretch (FIGURE 10-18)

• Lie down on your back.

• Your left leg is extended toward the ceiling.

• Your right leg is bent in toward your chest.

• Place your left hand on your right knee and your right hand on the outside of your right ankle.

• Your elbows stay wide and open.

Start the Single Leg Stretch

Step One (FIGURE 10-19)

• Inhale, bringing your chin to your chest. Lift your shoulders off of the mat. Come up as high as the base of your shoulder blades.

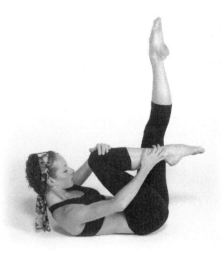

• Sink your navel toward your spine.

• Change legs and hands. This is **1 set.**

FIGURE 10-19

Step Two

• Exhale as you repeat.

Complete 3 to 5 sets.

Intermediate leg position:
- After you become strong enough, lower your extended leg closer toward the mat to approximately 60 degrees.

Prepare for the **Double Leg Stretch.**

DOUBLE LEG STRETCH

*This exercise will strengthen your Powerhouse
and enhance your coordination.*

SAFETY

Avoid lifting the head if you have neck problems.

THE VISUAL IMAGERY GUIDE

Centering
- Squeeze your buttocks and inner thighs together. **Picture a zipper fastening your heels, lower legs, upper legs, and buttocks together.**

- **Visualize spiraling your navel deep into the mat like a powerful whirlpool.**

- **Envision your ribcage wrapping tightly together as if you are wearing a corset.**

TEACHING TIPS

- Keep your head and shoulders raised throughout the exercise.

- Aim your legs toward the ceiling in order to "glue" your back into the mat.

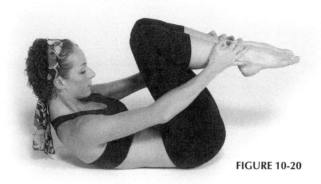

FIGURE 10-20

Preparation for the Double Leg Stretch (FIGURE 10-20)

• Lie on your back.

• Your legs are bent into your chest.

• Place your hands on your ankles.

• Bring your chin to your chest.

• Lift your shoulders off of the mat.

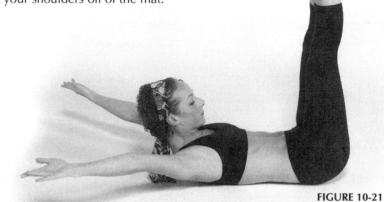

FIGURE 10-21

Start Double Leg Stretch

Step One (FIGURE 10-21)

• Inhale slowly as you stretch your arms back over your head.

• Your arms are in line with your ears.

• Simultaneously straighten your legs toward the ceiling.

• Slightly externally rotate your legs from the hip joints in the Pilates stance.

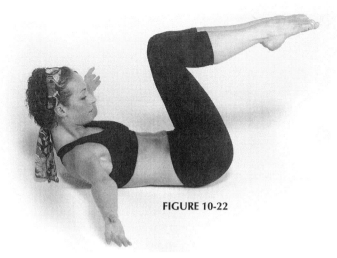

FIGURE 10-22

Step Two (FIGURE 10-22)

• Exhale as you sweep your arms out to your sides. Return your hands to your ankles as your legs bend into your chest.

Repeat 3-5 times.

TEACHING TIPS
Intermediate leg position: • When you are strong enough, lower your legs to approximately 60 degrees above the mat.

Prepare for the **Single Straight Leg Stretch**.

THE SINGLE STRAIGHT LEG STRETCH

This exercise stretches the back of the legs and strengthens the abdominal muscles.

SAFETY

Avoid lifting the head if you have neck problems. Skip this exercise if you have lower back problems.

THE VISUAL IMAGERY GUIDE

- Continuously scoop your navel in, back, and up.

- **Imagine anchoring your torso in heavy cement.**

- Stabilize your shoulder blades. **Glide them downward toward your back trouser pockets.**

TEACHING TIPS

- Hold your torso stable.

- Keep the neck and shoulders relaxed. Do not lift more than the base of your shoulders off of the mat.

- Depending on your flexibility, you may place your hands on the calf or back of the thigh. Do not hold behind the knee.

- It may be necessary to bend your knees.

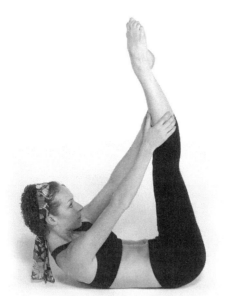

FIGURE 10-23

Preparation for Single Straight Leg Stretch

Step One (FIGURE 10-23)

• Lift your head and shoulders off the mat.

• Extend the legs toward the ceiling.

• Your hands reach toward the ankles.

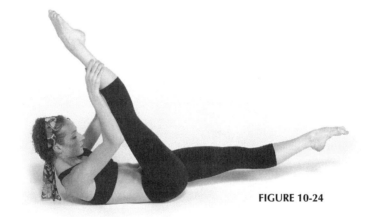

FIGURE 10-24

Start the Single Straight Leg Stretch

Step Two (FIGURE 10-24)

• Exhale while gently pulsing the top leg toward you twice, holding the ankle. Stretch the bottom leg out.

• Inhale, switching your legs in a "scissor" action. Breathe out to repeat the set.

Repeat 5-10 times.

Prepare for the **Double Straight Leg Stretch.**

THE DOUBLE STRAIGHT LEG STRETCH

This exercise works the Powerhouse.

SAFETY

Avoid if you have back problems. You may have the head down if you have a weak neck.

THE VISUAL IMAGERY GUIDE

• **Lower the legs slowly like a window shade closing, and raise the legs faster, opening the shade.** Use resistance to control the movement.

TEACHING TIPS

Place the hands behind your head. Layer one hand over the other without interlocking the fingers. The elbows stay wide. You may wish to straighten your arms by your sides.

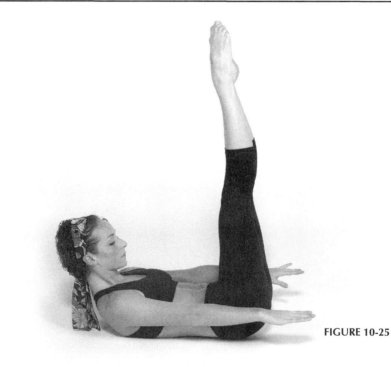

FIGURE 10-25

Preparation for Double Straight Leg Stretch (FIGURE 10-25)

• Sink your navel inward and bring your upper body up off the mat.

• Extend both legs straight up with the legs glued together. Externally rotate the legs in the Pilates stance.

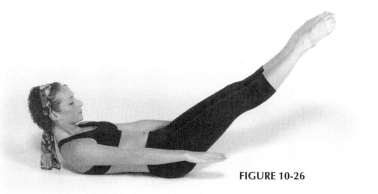

FIGURE 10-26

Start the Double Straight Leg Stretch

Step One (FIGURE 10-26)

• Inhale and slowly lower your legs about halfway to the mat.

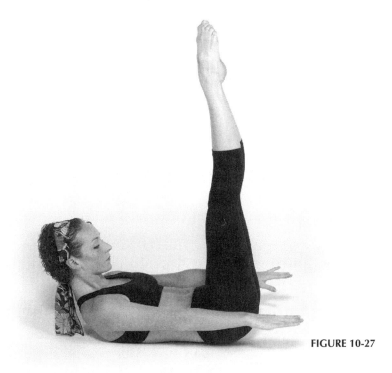

FIGURE 10-27

Step Two (FIGURE 10-27)

• Exhale and return your legs a bit faster to the starting position.

Finish

Repeat 5-10 times.

Bring both knees to your chest to prepare for **Crisscross**.

CRISSCROSS

This exercise targets the obliques to work the waist

SAFETY

Omit this exercise if you have a weak neck or back.

THE VISUAL IMAGERY GUIDE

- **Visualize a corkscrew spiraling each time you twist your body and hold for 3 counts.** During the 3 counts deepen the contraction of your abdominals to keep the trunk steady.

- **Picture tucking your shirt into trousers to organize your shoulder girdle**.

TEACHING TIPS

- Layer the hands behind your head without interlocking the fingers.

- Keep the elbows wide. Look at your back elbow when you twist.

- Hips remain stable.

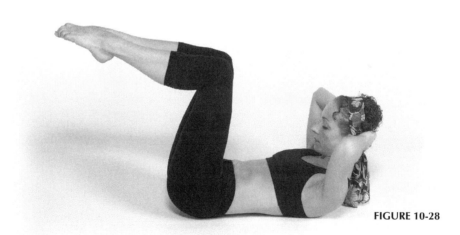

FIGURE 10-28

Preparation for Crisscross (FIGURE 10-28)
- Supine. Draw the knees into the body. Lift the upper body off the mat.

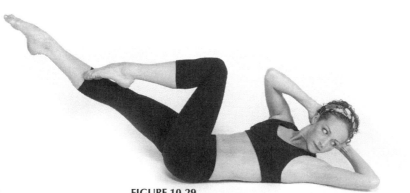

FIGURE 10-29

Step One (FIGURE 10-29)

• Straighten your right leg out at a 45-degree angle. Inhale, twist from your waistline. Bring your right elbow toward your left knee.

• Exhale, hold for 3 counts and deepen the abdominal contraction.

Step Two

• Inhale as you change to the other side.

Repeat 3-5 sets.

Finish

Master the exercises in this chapter before moving to the **Sports Mat Program**. Routinely perform the stretches in Chapter Nine for safety and success in your mat workouts.

Chapter Eleven

The Sports Mat Program

These are Pilates sports specific cross-training exercises. They enhance your overall level of fitness as well as your walking program, golf or tennis game, or any sport. These include intermediate and advanced level exercises that you can progress to after comfortably completing the **Basic Pilates Mat** exercises.

These exercises contain a mixture of spirals, circles, diagonals, and arcing pathways. They mimic many sports movements. Pilates sports conditioning exercises must focus upon moving the body into three-dimensional space. For example, a tennis player's service motion fills the space—back, up, and around the body. Define each movement orientation by *visualizing your body moving within a three-dimensional cube.* See yourself moving within this cube through *every* millimeter of these movements. Take up your vertical (up and down), horizontal (side to side), and sagittal (forward and back) space fully. Imagine you are a dancer performing on stage. Fill the three-dimensional space around your body with precision and conviction. Inspire the audience members seated in the last row of the theatre.

The **Sports Mat** exercises are about *intention*. Visual imagery draws out your inner dancer or athlete. Infuse each exercise with a commitment to sense every aspect of the movement. Take your time. Luxuriate in the sensations of moving your body. Picture the image in your mind while you physically implement it into your body. Explore the dynamics of *movement initiation* from the interior of your body outwards—and *then* move through space. These movements transport you to a feeling of freedom and joy.

The Foundation Exercise

SITTING TO C-CURVE WITH CORE CONTROL

Peak Performers: *Fitness Training, Dance, and the Martial Arts*

Sports Specific Cross Training: *All Sports*

Particularly for That Competitive Edge in Golf, Tennis, Skating, Gymnastics, and Fencing

THE VISUAL IMAGERY GUIDE

Centering
Visual Images: Jaw closing, corset, girdle, hug, and navel to spine.

IMAGINE YOUR ABDOMINALS CAN CONTRACT IN THE FOLLOWING WAYS FOR THE FIVE STEPS OF **The Foundation Exercise:**

Step One: **Jaw Closing**

Step Two: **Upper Corset**

Step Three: **Lower Girdle**

Step Four: **Hug**

Step Five: **Navel to Spine**

SAFETY

Omit this exercise if you have had recent back or abdominal problems.

Level: Beginner
This exercise is still very valuable sitting upright in "neutral."

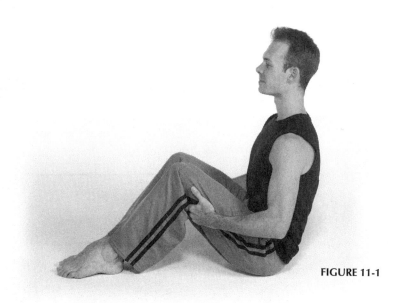

FIGURE 11-1

Position for The Foundation Exercise (FIGURE 11-1)

- Sit on the floor on a mat.

- Your knees are bent.

- The soles of your feet are firmly planted on the mat. Your heels are approximately two feet away from your hips.

- Your legs are pressed together.

- Wrap your hands behind your thighs.

- Draw your waistline in and up.

SUCCESS

NEVER LET YOUR ABDOMINALS RELAX BETWEEN THE FOLLOWING *FIVE* STEPS. Keep inwardly shaping them.

Your buttock, upper thigh, and pelvic floor muscles remain engaged.

Start The Foundation Exercise
Use your ABCs.

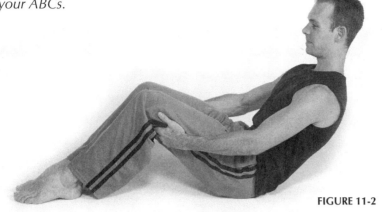

FIGURE 11-2

Step One: Jaw Closing

• Inhale fully. **(FIGURE 11-2)**

• Lengthen the sound of your exhale as you contract your abdominals. Curl back into a deep C-curve, behind your sit-bones. The back of your waistline aims at the floor.

• Look into your midsection.

THE VISUAL IMAGERY GUIDE FOR STEP ONE

• **This abdominal contraction feels like your ribcage and pubic bone draw together forcefully like a *jaw clamping shut*.**

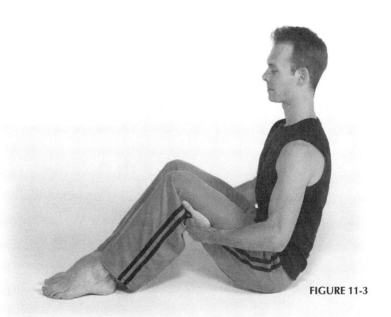

FIGURE 11-3

• Inhale as you sink your waist in deeper, returning to sitting. **(FIGURE 11-3)**

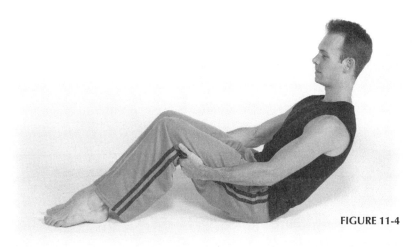

FIGURE 11-4

Step Two: Upper Corset (FIGURE 11-4)

• Exhale powerfully as you contract your abdominals, moving back again into your C-curve.

THE VISUAL IMAGERY GUIDE FOR STEP TWO

• This abdominal contraction feels like strings of a *corset* attached to the bottom of each one of your ribs. The strings are pulling inward and downward along the front of your body toward your hips.

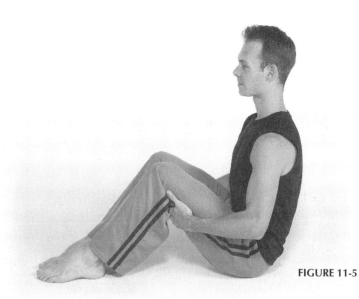

FIGURE 11-5

• Inhale as you keep the abdominals contracted, returning to sitting. **(FIGURE 11-5)**

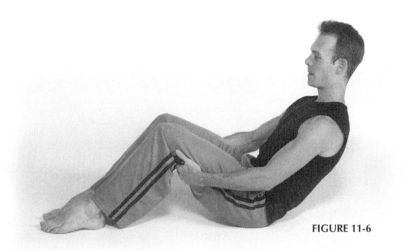

FIGURE 11-6

Step Three: Lower Girdle (FIGURE 11-6)

• Exhale forcefully as you contract your abdominals moving backwards into
your C-curve.

THE VISUAL IMAGERY GUIDE FOR STEP THREE

• **This feels like the powerful elastic action of a *lower girdle* drawing your
abdominal wall in, back, and up.** The center of your body takes on a
hollow, scooped-out bowl shape.

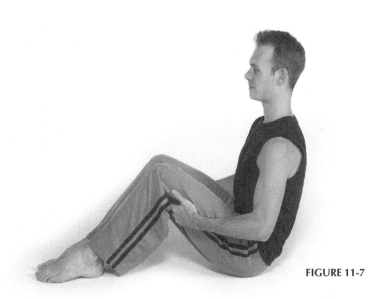

FIGURE 11-7

• Inhale as you contract your abdominals, returning to sitting. **(FIGURE 11-7)**

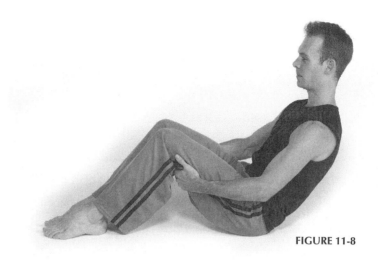

FIGURE 11-8

Step Four: Hug (FIGURE 11-8)

- Exhale strongly as you activate your abdominals, moving backwards into your C-curve.

THE VISUAL IMAGERY GUIDE FOR STEP FOUR

- **This abdominal contraction feels like a low seat belt being drawn together across your belly. Visualize that your abdominal muscle fibers can slide across each other like an *internal hug*.**

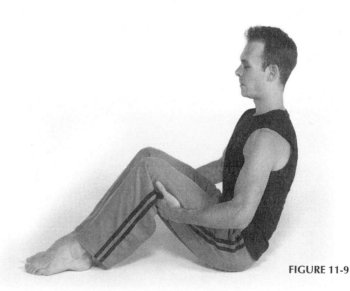

FIGURE 11-9

- Inhale keeping the abdominals engaged, returning to sitting. **(FIGURE 11-9)**

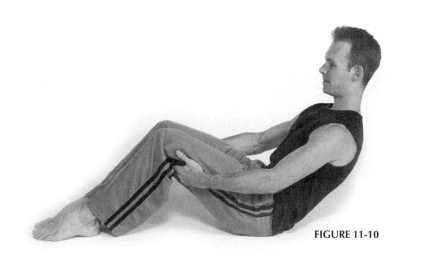

FIGURE 11-10

Step Five: Navel to Spine (FIGURE 11-10)

• Exhale as you contract your abdominal muscles, moving backwards into your C-curve.

THE VISUAL IMAGERY GUIDE FOR STEP FIVE

• **To feel this abdominal contraction visualize your shoulder girdle and ribcage are a shirt. Firmly tuck this shirt into your pants. Then fasten the belt of your pants tightly together at the waistline. Your belt *sinks your navel to your spine.***

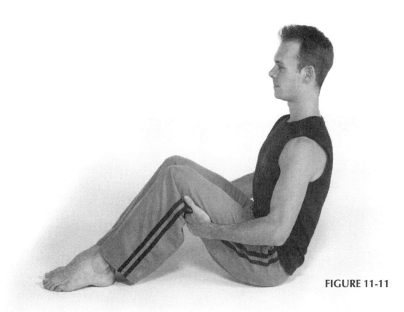

FIGURE 11-11

Finish The Foundation Exercise

• Inhale as you feel your abdominals going through to your backbone, returning to sitting. **(FIGURE 11-11)**

Repeat 3-5 times.

SUCCESS

Variation 1 of The Foundation Exercise

• When your abdominals are strong enough and do not shake, roll down all the way to supine. Exhale powerfully while moving. Perform the entire sequence of **The Foundation Exercise** while rolling down to supine. Say to yourself, ***"jaw closing, corset, girdle, hug, and navel to the spine"*** until you know the images from memory.

• Roll up one vertebra at a time to sitting. Perform the five steps of **The Foundation Exercise** while rolling up to sitting. Say, *"jaw-corset-girdle-hug-navel"* to yourself.

Variation 2 of The Foundation Exercise adding Arm Movements

Add arm movements to **The Foundation Exercise** that mimic the direction of the muscular lines of force for each layer of your abdominals.

Position: Sit with your legs bent and together. Your feet are flat on the floor.

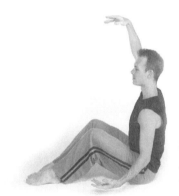

| FIGURE 11-12 | FIGURE 11-13 |

Start

Step One: Jaw Closing (FIGURE 11-12, 11-13)

Arms: One arm begins overhead; the other is low. As you move *backwards* into your C-curve, **the arms mimic a large mouth closing**. *Return to sitting*.

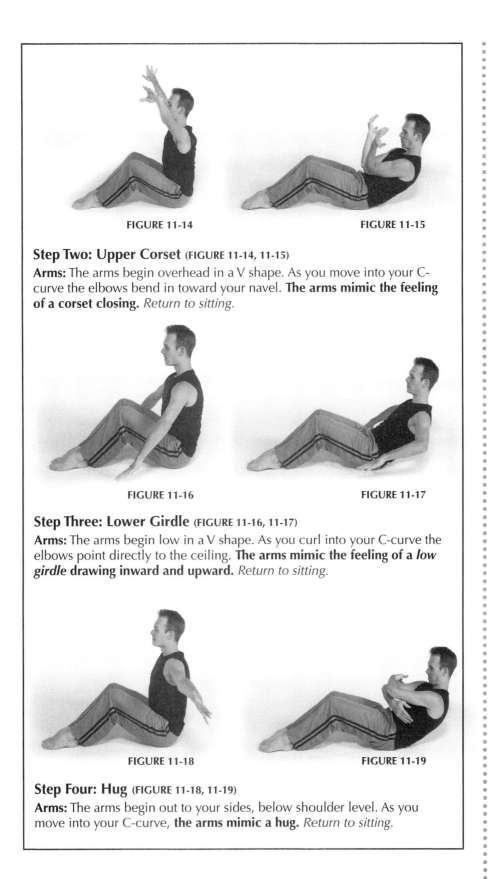

FIGURE 11-14   FIGURE 11-15

Step Two: Upper Corset (FIGURE 11-14, 11-15)

Arms: The arms begin overhead in a V shape. As you move into your C-curve the elbows bend in toward your navel. **The arms mimic the feeling of a corset closing.** *Return to sitting.*

FIGURE 11-16   FIGURE 11-17

Step Three: Lower Girdle (FIGURE 11-16, 11-17)

Arms: The arms begin low in a V shape. As you curl into your C-curve the elbows point directly to the ceiling. **The arms mimic the feeling of a *low girdle* drawing inward and upward.** *Return to sitting.*

FIGURE 11-18   FIGURE 11-19

Step Four: Hug (FIGURE 11-18, 11-19)

Arms: The arms begin out to your sides, below shoulder level. As you move into your C-curve, **the arms mimic a hug.** *Return to sitting.*

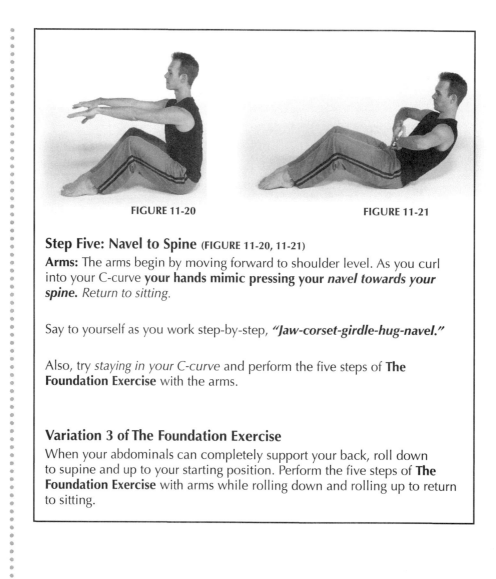

FIGURE 11-20   FIGURE 11-21

Step Five: Navel to Spine (FIGURE 11-20, 11-21)

Arms: The arms begin by moving forward to shoulder level. As you curl into your C-curve **your hands mimic pressing your *navel towards your spine.*** *Return to sitting.*

Say to yourself as you work step-by-step, ***"Jaw-corset-girdle-hug-navel."***

Also, try *staying in your C-curve* and perform the five steps of **The Foundation Exercise** with the arms.

Variation 3 of The Foundation Exercise

When your abdominals can completely support your back, roll down to supine and up to your starting position. Perform the five steps of **The Foundation Exercise** with arms while rolling down and rolling up to return to sitting.

Hug A Ball

SITTING TO C-CURVE ARMS HUG A BALL

Peak Performers: *Fitness Training, Dance*

Sports Specific Cross Training: *All Sports*

Particularly for That Competitive Edge In Basketball, Skating, and Surfing

THE VISUAL IMAGERY GUIDE

Hug a big imaginary ball with your arms and body. Your arms and trunk encircle a large volume of space. Picture ballet arms, which are extended but slightly curved.

FITNESS LEVELS

ALL

SAFETY

Omit this exercise if you have had recent back or abdominal problems.

Level: Beginner
Omit the C-curve. Stay sitting upright in "neutral."

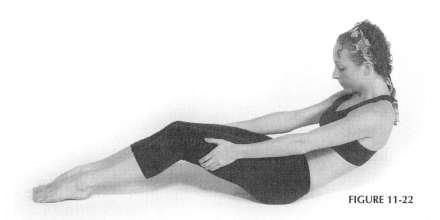

FIGURE 11-22

Position for Hug a Ball (FIGURE 11-22)
- Sit on the floor.

- Bend your knees with the soles of your feet planted firmly on the mat.

- Roll backwards off of your sit-bones into your deep C-curve.

Stay in the C-curve for the following arm movements:

Start Hug a Ball
Use your ABCs

Step One (FIGURE 11-23)
- Inhale.

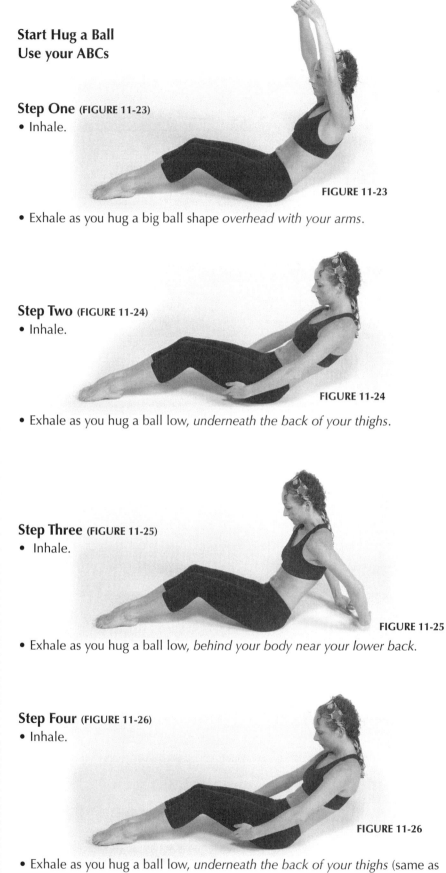

FIGURE 11-23

- Exhale as you hug a big ball shape *overhead with your arms*.

Step Two (FIGURE 11-24)
- Inhale.

FIGURE 11-24

- Exhale as you hug a ball low, *underneath the back of your thighs*.

Step Three (FIGURE 11-25)
- Inhale.

FIGURE 11-25

- Exhale as you hug a ball low, *behind your body near your lower back*.

Step Four (FIGURE 11-26)
- Inhale.

FIGURE 11-26

- Exhale as you hug a ball low, *underneath the back of your thighs* (same as Step Two).

Step Five (FIGURE 11-27)

- Inhale.

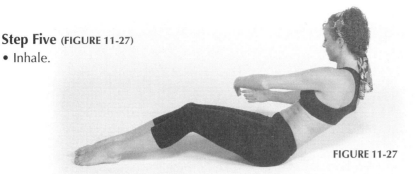

FIGURE 11-27

- Exhale as you hug a ball *diagonally, off of the right hip.*

Step Six (FIGURE 11-28)

- Inhale.

FIGURE 11-28

- Exhale as you hug a ball *diagonally, off of the left hip.*

Finish

- Return to sitting.

Repeat 3-5 times.

SUCCESS

Variation of Hug a Ball
Do this exercise when your abdominals are strong enough.

- *Perform the arm movements in steps one through six* while rolling all the way down to supine, and while returning to sitting.

- To remember the six arm positions for the **Hug a Ball** exercise say to yourself, *"Up, down, back, down, side, to side."*

Nautilus Shell

SITTING TO C-CURVE
LEG BENDS AND EXTENDS

Peak Performers: *Fitness Training, Dance*

Sports Specific Cross Training: *All Sports*

Particularly for That Competitive Edge in Skating, Swimming, Diving, and Gymnastics

THE VISUAL IMAGERY GUIDE

Nautilus shell. Visualize curling your body over a *large nautilus shell* when you move into your C-curve.

SAFETY

Omit this exercise if you have had recent back or abdominal problems. Avoid if you have had a hip replacement.

FITNESS LEVELS

ALL

THE PRINCIPLES OF MOVEMENT – ABCs

Alignment • Breathing Centering and Core Stability

Position for Nautilus Shell

• Sit with your knees bent and the soles of your feet firmly planted on the mat.

• Place your heels approximately two feet away from your hips.

Start Nautilus Shell
Use your ABCs.

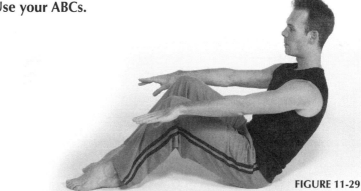

FIGURE 11-29

Step One (FIGURE 11-29)
• Inhale.

• Exhale as you roll backwards into your deep C-curve.

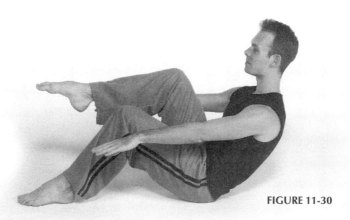

FIGURE 11-30

Step Two (FIGURE 11-30)

• Inhale as you *brush* your right foot backwards along the mat bringing your knee toward your chest.

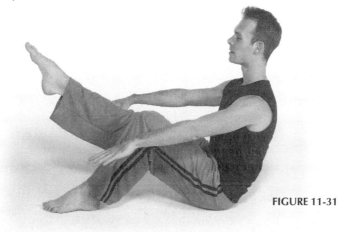

FIGURE 11-31

Finish (FIGURE 11-31)

• Exhale as you *brush* your right foot forward along the mat.

• Extend your leg while gradually returning to a sitting position.

Change legs.

Repeat 3-5 times.

SUCCESS

A Variation of Nautilus Shell
(FIGURE 11-32, 11-33)

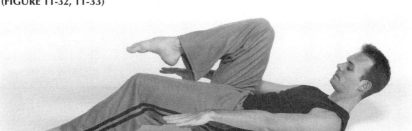

FIGURE 11-32

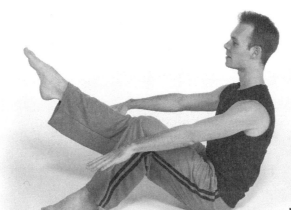

FIGURE 11-33

• When your abdominals are strong enough, roll backwards to supine.

• The gesture foot still *brushes along the mat* and the gesture leg bends into the chest as you roll down to supine.

• Return to sitting.

• While rolling up to sitting, the gesture foot *brushes along the mat* forward to a straight leg.

Change sides.

Repeat each leg 3-5 times.

Beats

SIT, LEANING BACKWARDS ON FOREARMS LEGS RHYTHMICALLY ABDUCT AND ADDUCT

Peak Performers: *Fitness Training, Dance*

Sports Specific Cross Training: *All Sports*

Particularly for That Competitive Edge in Football, Skating, Triple Jump, and Skiing

THE VISUAL IMAGERY GUIDE

Rhythmical scissoring motion of the legs.

SAFETY

Omit this exercise if you have had recent back or abdominal problems. Avoid supporting yourself on your arms if you have rotator cuff problems.

Level: Beginner
Bend your legs.

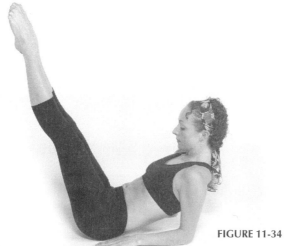

FIGURE 11-34

Position for Beats (FIGURE 11-34)

• Sit leaning back on your forearms.

• Lift your legs off of the mat. Extend your legs into the Pilates stance. Tighten your buttocks and squeeze the back of your upper inner thighs together. Your body and legs form a V shape. Keep your legs high. This is a good position for the lower back. The abdominals can be easily recruited and the pelvis is supported. Each time you exhale the abdominals contract deeper.

191

**Start Beats
Use your ABCs.**

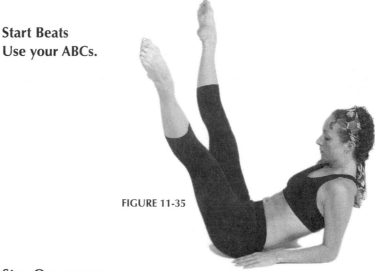

FIGURE 11-35

Step One (FIGURE 11-35)
• Inhale as you move your legs apart.

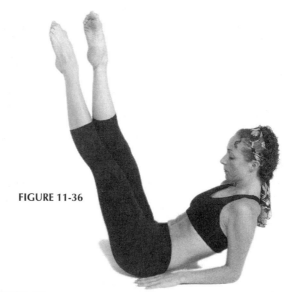

FIGURE 11-36

Step Two (FIGURE 11-36)
• Exhale as your ankles come together. Cross your right ankle in front of your left ankle.

Step Three
• Continue alternating which foot is in the front using a scissoring leg motion. In ballet these are called **beats**.

Repeat from 5-15 times.

You may also want to *hold or pause* the beating motion when your legs come together. This rhythm sounds like and ONE and TWO and…etc.

A Variation of Beats (FIGURE 11-37, 11-38)

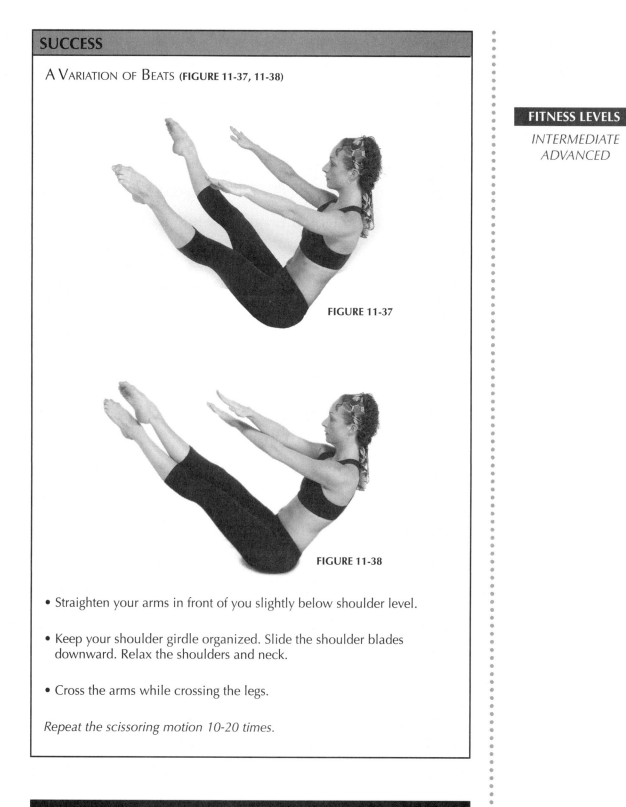

FIGURE 11-37

FIGURE 11-38

FITNESS LEVELS

*INTERMEDIATE
ADVANCED*

- Straighten your arms in front of you slightly below shoulder level.

- Keep your shoulder girdle organized. Slide the shoulder blades downward. Relax the shoulders and neck.

- Cross the arms while crossing the legs.

Repeat the scissoring motion 10-20 times.

SAFETY

Your abdominals must be very strong. Keep the motion slow and controlled. Your legs stay high to care for your lower back.

Coil

SUPINE
TRUNK FLEXION TO SITTING
ADD TRUNK ROTATION

Peak Performers: *Fitness Training, Dance*

Sports Specific Cross Training: *All Sports*

Particularly for That Competitive Edge in Golf, Tennis, Skiing, Discus, and Snowboarding

THE VISUAL IMAGERY GUIDE

Spiraling, winding, and looping. Imagine a coil being stretched and wound in two opposite directions.

SAFETY

Omit this exercise if you have abdominal, lower back, or thoracic problems.

Level: Beginner
If you are unable to roll up without distending the abdominals, perform the sitting rotation only. Keep your spine in "neutral."

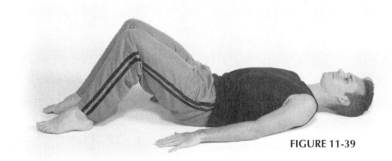

FIGURE 11-39

Position for Coil (FIGURE 11-39)
• Lie in supine on the mat.

• The legs are bent with the soles of your feet planted firmly on the mat. Your heels are approximately two feet away from your hips. Arms are by your sides.

Start Coil
Use your ABCs.

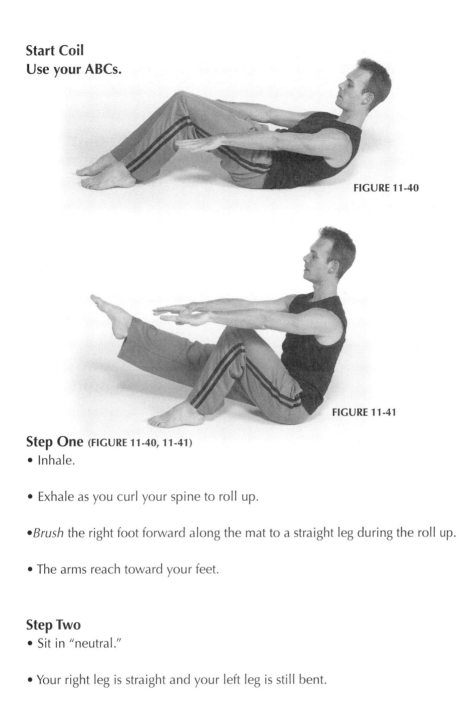

FIGURE 11-40

FIGURE 11-41

Step One (FIGURE 11-40, 11-41)

• Inhale.

• Exhale as you curl your spine to roll up.

•*Brush* the right foot forward along the mat to a straight leg during the roll up.

• The arms reach toward your feet.

Step Two

• Sit in "neutral."

• Your right leg is straight and your left leg is still bent.

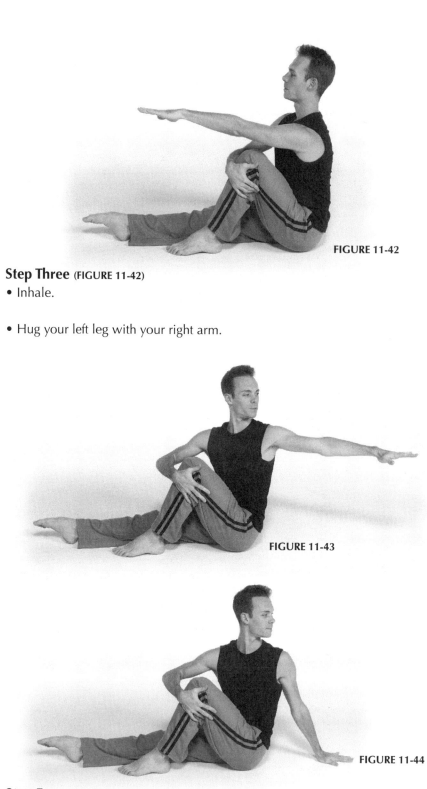

FIGURE 11-42

Step Three (FIGURE 11-42)

• Inhale.

• Hug your left leg with your right arm.

FIGURE 11-43

FIGURE 11-44

Step Four (FIGURE 11-43, 11-44)

• Exhale as you rotate your spine to the left. You are looking over your left shoulder. Place your left arm on the mat behind you. The hips remain facing forward.

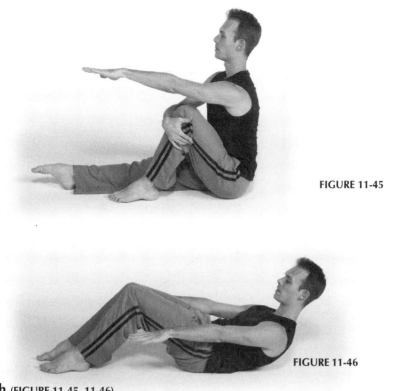

FIGURE 11-45

FIGURE 11-46

Finish (FIGURE 11-45, 11-46)

• Inhale as you come out of rotation.

• Exhale as you curl backwards into a C-curve returning to supine.

Change sides.

Repeat each side 3-5 times.

Wave

SUPINE BRIDGING WITH HIP ROTATION

Peak Performers: *Fitness Training, Dance*

Sports Specific Cross Training: *All Sports*

Particularly for That Competitive Edge in Rock Climbing, Baseball, Tennis, Skiing, and Equestrian Events

THE VISUAL IMAGERY GUIDE

An ocean wave lapping in and out over the shoreline. Imagine that when your abdominals contract they move toward your head on your inhales and toward your feet on your exhales. Visualize *waves* washing across the shoreline and back out again.

SAFETY

Omit this exercise if you have hip, abdominal, or back problems.

Level: Beginner
Omit the rotation of the hips.

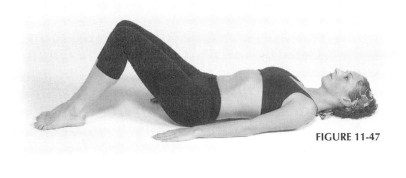

FIGURE 11-47

Position for Wave (FIGURE 11-47)

• Lie down on your back.

• Bend your knees with the soles of your feet planted firmly on the mat.

198

**Start Wave
Use your ABCs.**

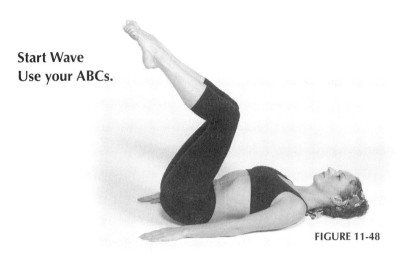

FIGURE 11-48

Step One (FIGURE 11-48)

• Inhale as you bring the knees toward your chest.

Step Two

• Exhale as you gently stomp both feet back onto the mat.

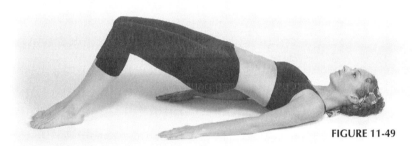

FIGURE 11-49

Step Three (FIGURE 11-49)

• Inhale.

• Exhale as you slowly raise your hips off of the mat. Do this by successively peeling one vertebra up off of the mat at a time. Begin with curling the tailbone, then the sacrum, the back of the waistline, and the ribcage off of the mat. Pilates refers to this as "bridging" or "hinging."

• End supported on your shoulder blades.

Step Four

• Place a hand on each of your hipbones. This will help guide the next movement.

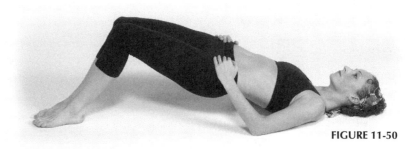

FIGURE 11-50

Step Five (FIGURE 11-50)

- Inhale as you rotate both of your hipbones toward the left. This is a small rotational movement, approximately 1 inch.

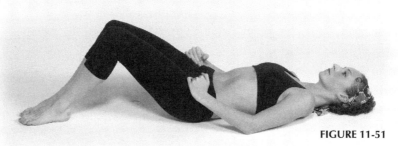

FIGURE 11-51

Finish (FIGURE 11-51)

- Exhale as you remain in rotation; slowly roll back down through the vertebrae of the spine. Begin with the ribcage, waistline, and sacrum, and finally the tailbone lands on the mat. You will gradually end with your pelvis back in the center position you began in.

THE VISUAL IMAGERY GUIDE
Imagine your back can spread across the mat like sand being flattened by a *wave* on your way back down to supine.

Change to the other side.

Repeat 3-5 times.

FITNESS LEVELS

INTERMEDIATE
ADVANCED

SUCCESS

A Variation of Wave
Perform Wave with a single leg.

Position
Lying down with the knees bent, and the arms by your sides.

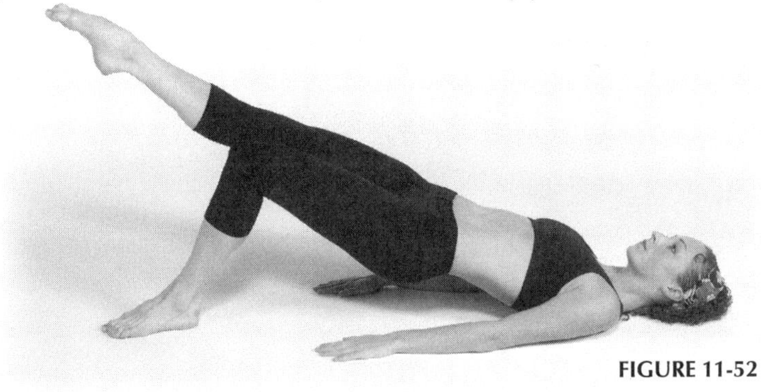

FIGURE 11-52

Start (FIGURE 11-52)

- Lift both legs toward your chest. Gently stomp both feet onto the mat. After the stomp, your right gesture leg straightens. It attaches *thigh against thigh* to your left support leg.

- Move into your hinge position supported by your left leg only. End by resting on your shoulder blades. *The hips turn to the left when you support on your left leg and vice versa.* Roll back down one vertebra at a time. As your tail bone lands both feet are placed flat on the floor. Change sides. *Repeat 3-5 times.*

Crescent Moon

PRONE
WITH TRUNK EXTENSION

Peak Performers: *Fitness Training, Dance, and Yoga*

Sports Specific Cross Training: *All Sports*

Particularly for That Competitive Edge in High Jumping, Swimming, Diving, Gymnastics, and Skating

FITNESS LEVELS

ALL

THE VISUAL IMAGERY GUIDE

Crescent moon shape. Imagine your body lengthening in two opposite directions, like a *crescent moon.*

SAFETY

Omit this exercise if you have back or rotator cuff problems.

Level: Beginners
- Perform with your hands placed beneath your shoulder joints.

- Your forearms will remain on the floor.

- Omit the arm circles.

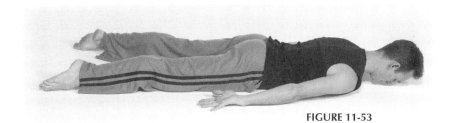

FIGURE 11-53

Position for Crescent Moon (FIGURE 11-53)
- Prone. Your arms are by your sides. Your legs are externally rotated. Tighten your buttocks and squeeze your legs together.

**Start Crescent Moon
Use your ABCs.**

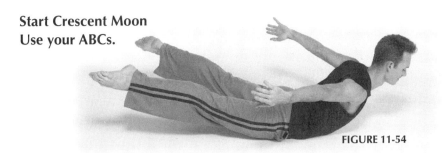

FIGURE 11-54

Step One (FIGURE 11-54)

• Inhale.

• Exhale, sliding your shoulder blades toward your hips, as you rise slowly into spine extension.

• Your upper body will only lift four to six inches away from the mat.

• *Your gaze stays down so that the back of your neck stays long.*

• Lengthen your legs away from your head making a shallow crescent moon shape with your body. The legs can remain on the mat.

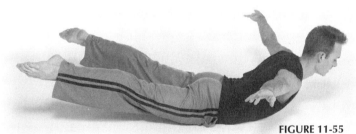

FIGURE 11-55

Step Two (FIGURE 11-55)

• Inhale.

• Exhale as your arms trace one small circle out to your sides.

Finish

• Inhale as you return to the mat.

Repeat 3 times.

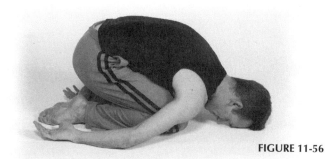

FIGURE 11-56

CURL INTO THE **CHILD POSE** FROM YOGA: **(FIGURE 11-56)**
- The body is in a low kneeling posture.

- The trunk is folded over the legs.

- The head rests toward the floor.

- The arms are by your sides.

SUCCESS

A Variation of Crescent Moon
- Begin as above.

- Make three small circles of the arms in one direction. The arms are straight and out to your sides.

- Make three small circles of the arms in the other direction.

Bow

ON ALL FOURS
WITH CORE CONTROL
"NEUTRAL" SPINE AND TRUNK FLEXION
ONE LEG BENDS AND EXTENDS

Peak Performers: *Fitness Training, Dance, and Weight Training*

Sports Specific Cross Training: *All Sports*

Particularly for That Competitive Edge in Golf, Track and Field, Rock Climbing, and Fencing

THE VISUAL IMAGERY GUIDE

Bowing posture. Imagine a graceful *bow* in which your back arches like a cat stretching.

SAFETY

Omit this exercise if you have knee, lower back, or hip problems.

Level: Beginner
• Curl your trunk only. This is called the Cat in yoga.

• Omit lifting the leg.

You may want to practice using one arm only.

Position for Bow (FIGURE 11-57)
• Kneel on all fours.

• The hands are placed underneath the shoulder joints.

• The knees are placed underneath the hip joints.

• The back is in "neutral."

• The elbows are straight but not locked.

• The head is level and the eyes are focused directly in between your hands.

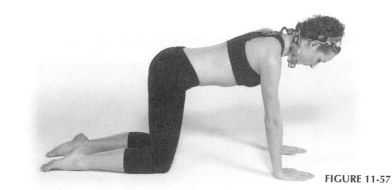

FIGURE 11-57

Start Bow
Use your ABCs.

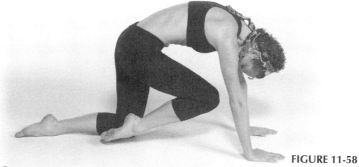

FIGURE 11-58

Step One (FIGURE 11-58)

• Inhale.

• Exhale as you curl your back into spine flexion. This looks like a cat arching its back. Bring your right knee toward your chest.

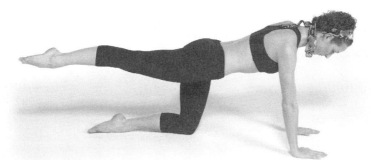

Step Two (FIGURE 11-59)

FIGURE 11-59

• Inhale.

• Exhale as you straighten your right leg behind you.

• Your back returns to "neutral."

Change sides.

Repeat 3-5 times.

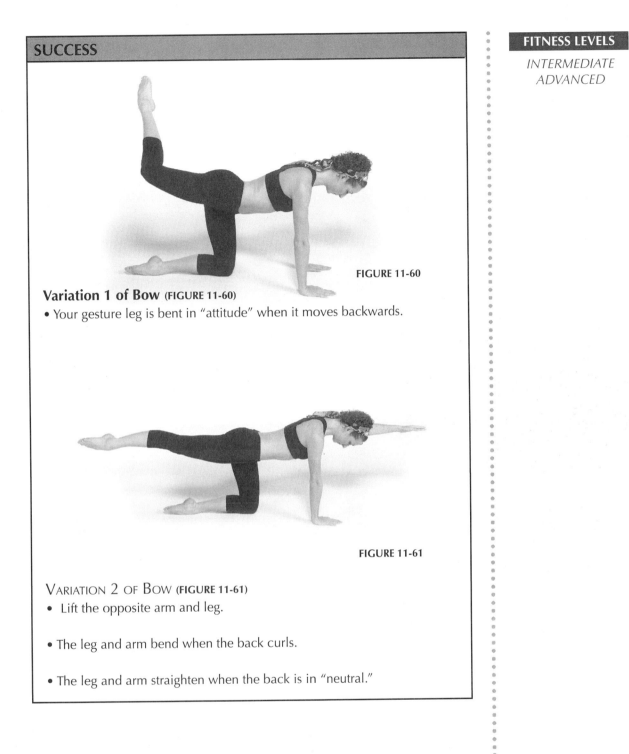

FIGURE 11-60

Variation 1 of Bow (FIGURE 11-60)

• Your gesture leg is bent in "attitude" when it moves backwards.

FIGURE 11-61

VARIATION 2 OF BOW (FIGURE 11-61)

• Lift the opposite arm and leg.

• The leg and arm bend when the back curls.

• The leg and arm straighten when the back is in "neutral."

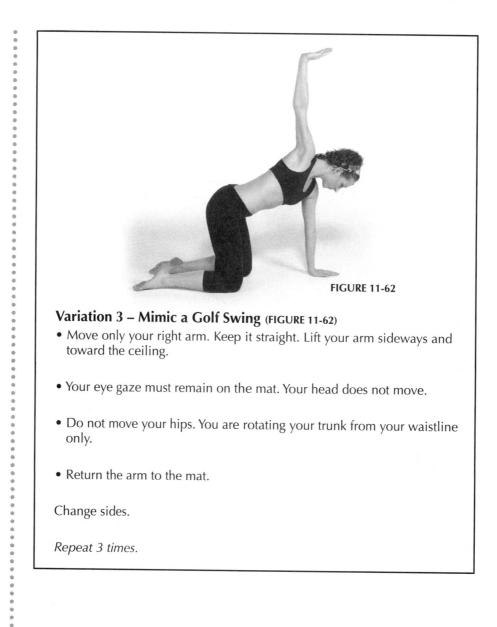

FIGURE 11-62

Variation 3 – Mimic a Golf Swing (FIGURE 11-62)

• Move only your right arm. Keep it straight. Lift your arm sideways and toward the ceiling.

• Your eye gaze must remain on the mat. Your head does not move.

• Do not move your hips. You are rotating your trunk from your waistline only.

• Return the arm to the mat.

Change sides.

Repeat 3 times.

Octopus

Z-SIT
WITH LATERAL FLEXION TO LYING ON YOUR SIDE

Peak Performers: *Fitness Training, Dance*

Sports Specific Cross Training: *All Sports*

Particularly for That Competitive Edge in Baseball, Swimming, Water Skiing, Ski Jumping, Skateboarding, Gymnastics, and Skating

THE VISUAL IMAGERY GUIDE

An octopus propelling itself. Imagine an *octopus* thrusting through the water from its center out through to its tentacles.

SAFETY

Omit this exercise if you have had a hip replacement or lower back problems.

Level - Beginner
If it is uncomfortable to Z-sit, perform the following exercise only:

- "Lounge" in Z-sit. Place your forearms or hands on the mat behind your body. Turn both of your knees from side to side.

Position for Octopus (FIGURE 11-63)

- Z-sit on the mat. In Z-sit, the legs are bent to the right side of your body. Your left foot is against your right knee.

- The arms are by your sides.

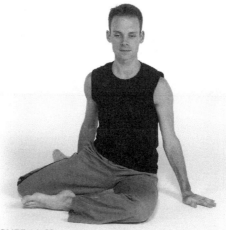

FIGURE 11-63

**Start Octopus
Use your ABCs.**

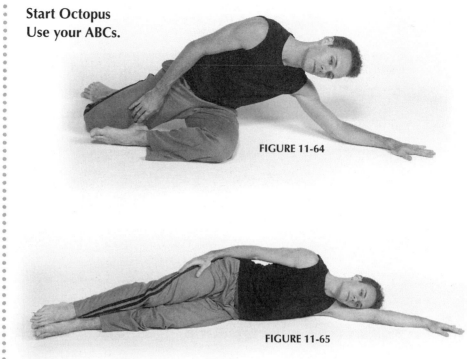

FIGURE 11-64

FIGURE 11-65

Step One (FIGURE 11-64, 11-65)

• Inhale.

• Exhale, curling down until you are lying on your left side. Your left arm slides along the floor.

• Gradually straighten your legs.

• The body ends in a stretched out position. Your legs are slightly in front of your hips.

Finish

• Inhale. Exhale as you curl up sideways until you are sitting in Z-sit.

Repeat 3-5 times.

Change Sides.

Variations of Octopus

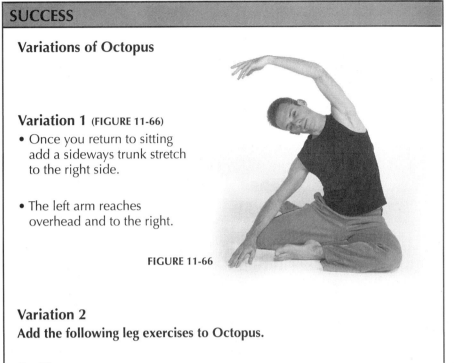

Variation 1 (FIGURE 11-66)

- Once you return to sitting add a sideways trunk stretch to the right side.

- The left arm reaches overhead and to the right.

FIGURE 11-66

Variation 2
Add the following leg exercises to Octopus.

Position

- From Z-sit, roll down until you are lying on your side. Align your body from your head to your hips.

- Your legs are slightly in front of your hips.

- Extend your bottom arm along the mat and rest your head on it.

- Your top arm is bent. The forearm is close to your waistline. The palm of your hand is flat on the mat.

Perform 3-5 repetitions of each of the following leg variations:

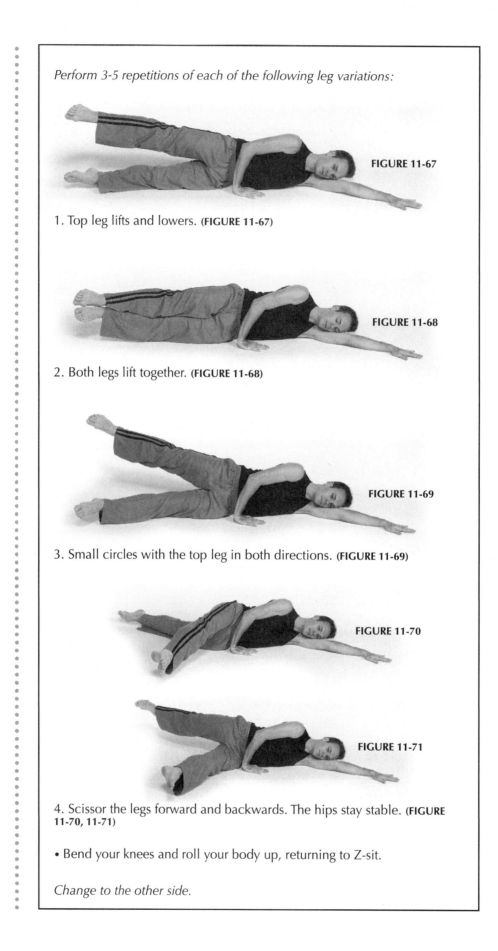

FIGURE 11-67

1. Top leg lifts and lowers. **(FIGURE 11-67)**

FIGURE 11-68

2. Both legs lift together. **(FIGURE 11-68)**

FIGURE 11-69

3. Small circles with the top leg in both directions. **(FIGURE 11-69)**

FIGURE 11-70

FIGURE 11-71

4. Scissor the legs forward and backwards. The hips stay stable. **(FIGURE 11-70, 11-71)**

• Bend your knees and roll your body up, returning to Z-sit.

Change to the other side.

Spiral

Z-SIT
WITH TRUNK AND HIP ROTATION

Peak Performers: *Fitness Training, Dance*

Sports Specific Cross Training: *All Sports*

Particularly for That Competitive Edge in Golf, Tennis, Basketball, Javelin, and Discus

THE VISUAL IMAGERY GUIDE

Rotating and spiraling in opposite directions. Imagine *spiraling* in two directions like a rag being wrung out.

SAFETY

Omit this exercise if you have hip, shoulder, or lower back problems.

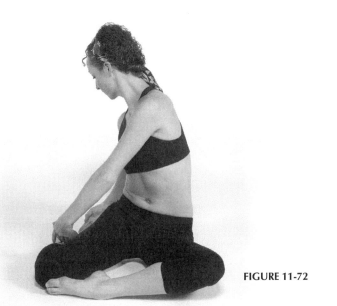

FIGURE 11-72

Position for Spiral (FIGURE 11-72)

- Z-sit on the mat. In Z-sit, your legs are bent toward the right side of your hips. Your left foot is against your right knee.

- Your arms and spine are rotated toward the right side of your hips.

- You are gazing over your right shoulder, toward the back corner of the room.

213

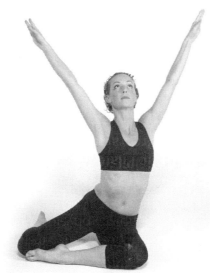

FIGURE 11-73

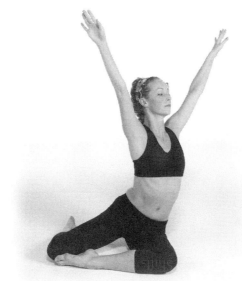

FIGURE 11-74

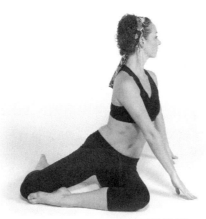

FIGURE 11-75

**Start Spiral
Use your ABCs.**

Step One
(FIGURE 11-73, 11-74, 11-75)

• Inhale.

• Exhale as you initiate a
rotation from your right
hipbone. The right side
of your hip lifts off of the
mat.

• Rotate your spine to the
left.

• The arms straighten
tracing an arcing pathway
overhead. Stabilize your
shoulder blades. Gently
slide them toward your
hips.

•The hands end on the mat
behind the left side of
your hips. You are gazing
over your left shoulder,
toward the back corner of
the room.

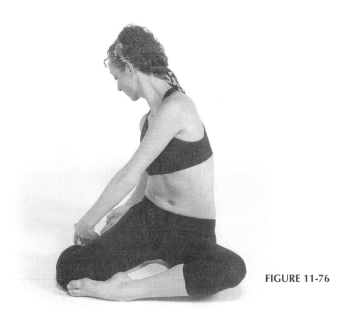

FIGURE 11-76

Finish (FIGURE 11-76)
- Inhale.

- Exhale as you return in the same way to the starting position.

FITNESS LEVELS

ALL

SUCCESS

Success
A Variation of Spiral

Variation 1

Position
- Z-sit on the mat. Your legs are bent toward the right side of your hips. Your left foot is against your right knee.

- Your arms and spine are rotated toward the right side of your hips.

- You are gazing over your right shoulder.

Start
- The right side of your hip lifts off of the mat. Initiate the spine rotation from your right hipbone.

- Rotate your spine to the left.

- The arms trace an arcing pathway overhead. Stabilize your shoulder blades. Gently slide them toward your hips.

- The hands end on the mat behind the left side of your hips.

- You are gazing over your left shoulder.

- Your weight is on the left side of your hip and outer thigh.

- Your right leg may either be bent or straight.

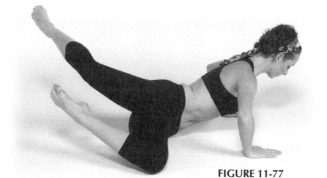

FIGURE 11-77

- Perform *sideways-facing* pushups on both hands. Bend and straighten your elbows. The body moves in one unit. **(FIGURE 11-77)**

- The legs remain in a low, stationary position. You may leave the legs on the mat. Increase the challenge with the legs hovering off of the mat.

Return to the starting position.

Variation 2 of Spiral

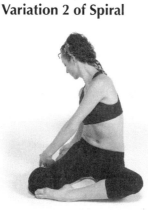

FIGURE 11-78

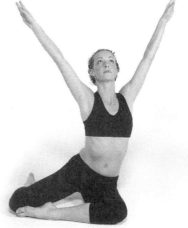

FIGURE 11-79

The exercise begins in the same way as **Variation 1** of the **Spiral** above. **(FIGURE 11-78)**

- The arms trace an arcing pathway overhead. **(FIGURE 11-79)**

- Place the left hand on the floor near your left hip.

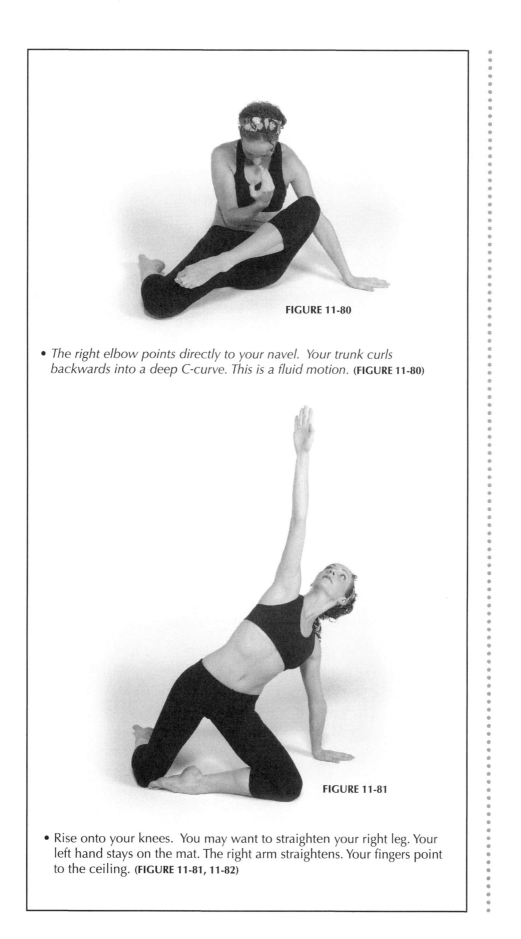

FIGURE 11-80

• *The right elbow points directly to your navel. Your trunk curls backwards into a deep C-curve. This is a fluid motion.* **(FIGURE 11-80)**

FIGURE 11-81

• Rise onto your knees. You may want to straighten your right leg. Your left hand stays on the mat. The right arm straightens. Your fingers point to the ceiling. **(FIGURE 11-81, 11-82)**

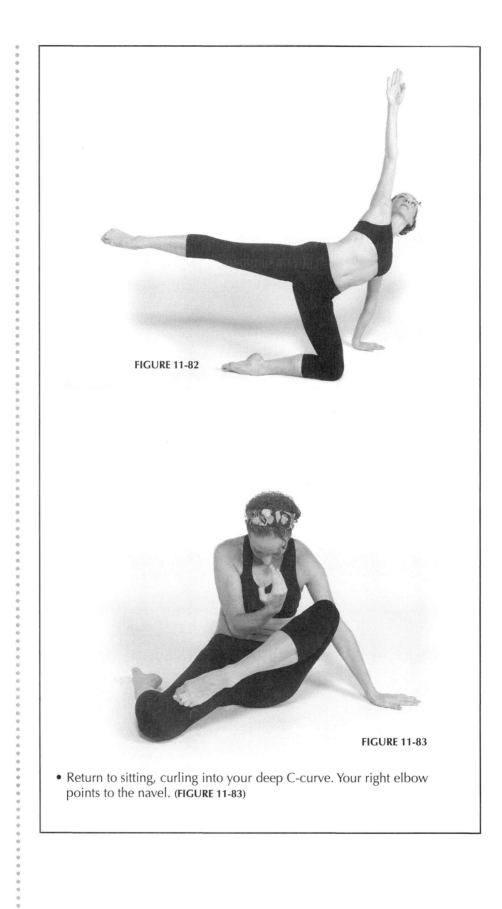

FIGURE 11-82

FIGURE 11-83

- Return to sitting, curling into your deep C-curve. Your right elbow points to the navel. **(FIGURE 11-83)**

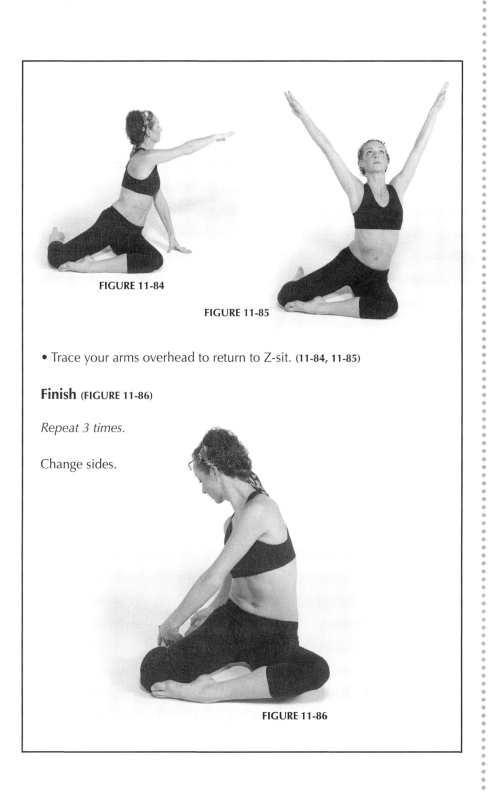

FIGURE 11-84

FIGURE 11-85

• Trace your arms overhead to return to Z-sit. **(11-84, 11-85)**

Finish (FIGURE 11-86)

Repeat 3 times.

Change sides.

FIGURE 11-86

Sports Mat Reference

The following contains information about your sports specific cross-training mat program in Chapter Eleven. The exercises enhance performance in all of your sports. Pilates is primarily *Functional Training*. The focus is on deep core strength, stabilization, and muscle isolation. This makes it the perfect complement to sports conditioning.

The **Sports Mat Program** combines scientific fitness training with an artistic component. This makes the exercises both functional and expressive. This fitness program is a blend of Pilates, sports, and dance movements. It includes components from dance such as visual imagery and three-dimensional movements through space. Visual imagery helps you reach and fire muscles that you never thought you had. Three-dimensional movements allow you to reach into space in ways that are unexplored in your daily activities. These components help you to access the artistry, inspiration, and joy of moving present in dance training.

Challenge yourself with these exercises after comfortably completing your **Basic Pilates Mat Program** in Chapter Ten. Those already doing Pilates can add these exercises to attain more coordination, speed, power, and range of motion.

The AthleticKinetic Recipe™ Cards

Principles of Movement—ABCs

INGREDIENTS

- Alignment
- Breathing
- Centering

METHOD

Mix the Principles of Movement to *clarify* the fundamentals of how the body functions. They are like a *well-stocked pantry*. This is the key to success for any fitness participant. The Sports Mat Program increases the Pilates challenge without compromising the principles.

Rudolf Laban's Elements of Movement

INGREDIENTS

Time	Attitude	Fast $\longleftrightarrow$	Slow
Space	Quality	Planes	Directions
		Levels	Pathways
Force	Weight	Heavy $\longleftrightarrow$	Light
	Effort	Strong $\longleftrightarrow$	Soft
Shape	Design	Round $\longleftrightarrow$	Pointed
		Large $\longleftrightarrow$	Small
Flow	Energy	Free $\longleftrightarrow$	Bound

METHOD

Stir in the delicious Elements that bring out the *qualities* of a movement. The Elements extend your movement possibilities. Reawaken muscles and joints not used in everyday movements. The emphasis is on total-body, spatial exploration rather than isolated body parts. The body moves as an efficient unit through three-dimensional space to enhance peak performance. Sports-specific cross-training programs require more spatial options—the areas behind the body (tennis, basketball), diagonal pathways and movements that cross the body (golf, skiing), twists, turns, spirals, circles, and rotational movements (gymnastics, skating). The focus is on three-dimensional mobility not sheer muscular strength.

The Moving Body's Relationship to Kinetics

Kinetics, noun: scientific study of forces and energy on the moving body. Adjective: Example: "Modern dance has been called kinetic pantomime."

INGREDIENTS

Gravity $\longleftrightarrow$ The Body $\longleftrightarrow$ Energy

Contraction $\longleftrightarrow$ Release

Balance $\longleftrightarrow$ Weight Shifts

Rhythm

Controlled Momentum

METHOD

Simmer:
Add the remaining *spicy* **Kinetics** to draw out the artistry and joy of movement. These essential ingredients create a greater potential for achieving peak performance.

Serving suggestion: Participants in fitness, sports, dance, yoga, martial arts, performance arts, and acrobatics. Pilates instructors, fitness trainers, coaches, movement therapists, physical therapists, dance teachers, and yoga teachers.

Recommendations: Complete the **Basic Pilates Mat Exercises** before progressing to the **Sports Mat Program.**

The World's Greatest Athletes Share the Artistry of Dancers

Sports Mat Program Recipe

The Moving Body's Relationship to Kinetic Energy

INGREDIENTS

Gravity $\longleftrightarrow$ The Body $\longleftrightarrow$ Energy

Contraction $\longleftrightarrow$ Release

Balance $\longleftrightarrow$ Weight Shifts

Rhythm

Controlled Momentum

In the practice of Pilates, you ideally feel the joy dancing brings to the spirit. The body moves with precision into all of the space around the body. The **Sports Mat exercises** help you experience an exhilarating combination of teetering, off-center, yet controlled movements. The **Sports Mat Program** began as an experiment with kinetics. Kinetics relate to the **energetic balance** between the **body's muscular contractions, weight shifts** and the **force of gravity**—resulting in a dance-like sensation of **controlled momentum**. Precise spiraling movements and changing **rhythms** complete this dance-inspired sports conditioning program.

Performance-level athletes have achieved the necessary technical prowess for their sport due to advancements in training. Today's athletes have to stand out artistically. This gives them that extra edge in order to win.

Elite athletes dive into the void with complete faith and love for extending movement vistas. They appear to control the reins of gravity. A snowboard jumper in one maneuver can do several complex flips and then land aligned—making it all look effortless. Any athlete or fitness enthusiast can acquire a more artistic dimension through the **Sports Mat Program**, along with a routine practice of the **Alignment, Breathing, and Centering** exercises. These exercises reinforce the guiding **principles of movement**. Including them into sports warm-ups, conditioning, and actual athletic events helps you soar past competitors.

Athletic skills can become art in motion using this challenging training. These dynamic exercises encompass the very *kinetic* foundation of dance expression. This is the *constant awareness* between the body's internal state of *muscular tension* and the external *force of gravity*.

Sometimes we can't keep our eyes off of a specific dancer. The "feeling dancer" who can maintain this *constant awareness* mesmerizes us more than the "flashy, technical virtuoso."

The technical dancer stays rooted in the physical body, appearing static, mechanical, and over-polished. The feeling dancer gives into the excitement of authentic spontaneity and the vitality of the continuous flow of motion, uplifting us artistically and spiritually.

Athletes and fitness participants can gain this dancer's *awareness*. They can initiate movements from their core trunk muscles. This inward shaping through deep abdominal muscular contractions stokes an athlete's engine. Their movements have more outward force. The body becomes moving sculpture.

The dancer has choreography; an athlete is always improvising. For example, the athlete's terrain, opponents, and weather change. This program's mind-body training addresses these continual adjustments in balance, rhythm, and controlled momentum.

Athletes are rewarded with a seamless mix of technical skill and artistry in performance. Fitness enthusiasts of all levels attain more results through a focus upon creative expression.

Sports Mat Program Recipe

Rudolf Laban's Elements of Movement

INGREDIENTS

Time	Attitude	Fast ⟵⟶ Slow	
Space	Quality	Planes	Directions
		Levels	Pathways
Effort	Force	Heavy ⟵⟶ Light	
		Strong ⟵⟶ Soft	
Shape	Design	Round ⟵⟶ Pointed	
		Large ⟵⟶ Small	
Flow	Energy	Free ⟵⟶ Bound	

Before coming to America, Joseph Pilates worked with the European pioneers of movement but he was closest with Rudolf Laban. His exercise method gained favor in the dance community primarily through Laban. Joseph learned more from him about how we move our body. Rudolf Laban (1879-1958) was a dancer, architect, and movement analyst who founded the clear language of the **Elements of Movement**. He referred to them as **time, space, effort, shape, and flow.**

His theories of the body and its relationship to effort and space have been affecting such fields as dance, sports, fitness, movement therapy, physical rehabilitation, psychology, corporate management, and creative dance for children.

Laban participated in the major European artistic activities of his time such as the development of modern dance. He also created Labanotation. It is an intricate notation system for movement, much like the notation of music. It is used primarily to record dance choreography. Every time we move we use each of Laban's **Elements**.

USE OF SPACE IN THE SPORTS MAT PROGRAM

The **Sports Mat Program** varies **spatial planes, directions, levels, and pathways** within a single exercise. For example, diagonal movements that cross the body are important to many sports such as golf, basketball, and skiing.

USE OF TIME IN THE SPORTS MAT PROGRAM

The majority of traditional Pilates exercises coincide with the even timing of the participant's breathing cycle. This consistent rhythm helps to provide deep abdominal support. The **Sports Mat Program** modifies the **Element** of **time** to add percussive accents. This sense of rhythm enhances coordination and speed, essential for sports.

USE OF FLOW IN THE SPORTS MAT PROGRAM

Pilates is mainly performed with a **bound flow energy** that is slow and controlled like the movements of T'ai Chi. The **Sports Mat Program** adds controlled **free flow** movements to relate more directly to sports' multi-functional use of energy. Exercises to enhance sports performance must utilize a wide range of energy, from feather-like softness to powerful bursts.

Your whole movement perspective changes when you become aware of the **Principles, Elements, and Kinetic components of Movement** during your **Sports Mat** workouts. An intellectual understanding of movement deepens your kinesthetic feel for an exercise—you attain your fitness goals.

Anatomical Charts

In Pilates, sports, and dance it is useful to know the muscles and general bone landmarks that are involved in various movements. It is helpful to know both the scientific and the layman's term. This reference can help you understand how your body works for safety and results.

Muscles

(FRONT VIEW)
The deep muscles are not shown

Scientific Term	Layman's Term
1 Biceps Brachii	*(biceps, bi's, guns)*
2 Pectoralis Major	*(chest, pecs)*
3 Serratus Anterior	
4 Rectus Abdominis	*(stomach, abdomen, abs, six pack, washboard, structural muscles)*
5 External Obliques	*(obliques, waist muscles, love handles)*
6 Internal Obliques	*(obliques)*
7 Transversus Abdominis	*(core stabilizers, deep postural abdominals, functional muscles)*
8 Iliopsoas: Psoas Major, Iliacus	*(psoas, hip flexors)*
9 Multifidus	
10 Quadriceps Femoris:	*(thigh, quads)*
11 Adductors	*(inner thigh, groin)*
12 Abductors	*(outer thigh)*
13 Tensor fasciae latae	*(T.F.L.)*
14 Iliotibial Band	*(T band)*
15 Tibialis anterior	*(shin muscles, front of the lower leg)*

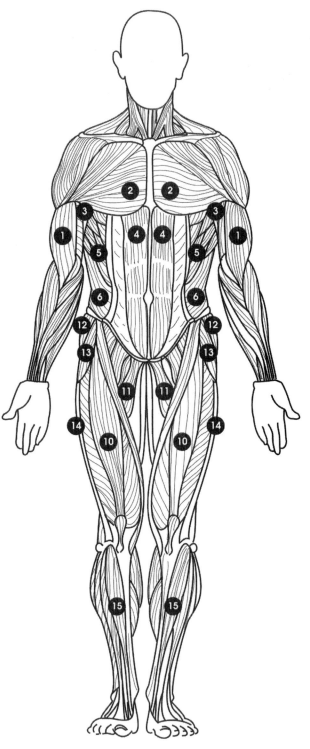

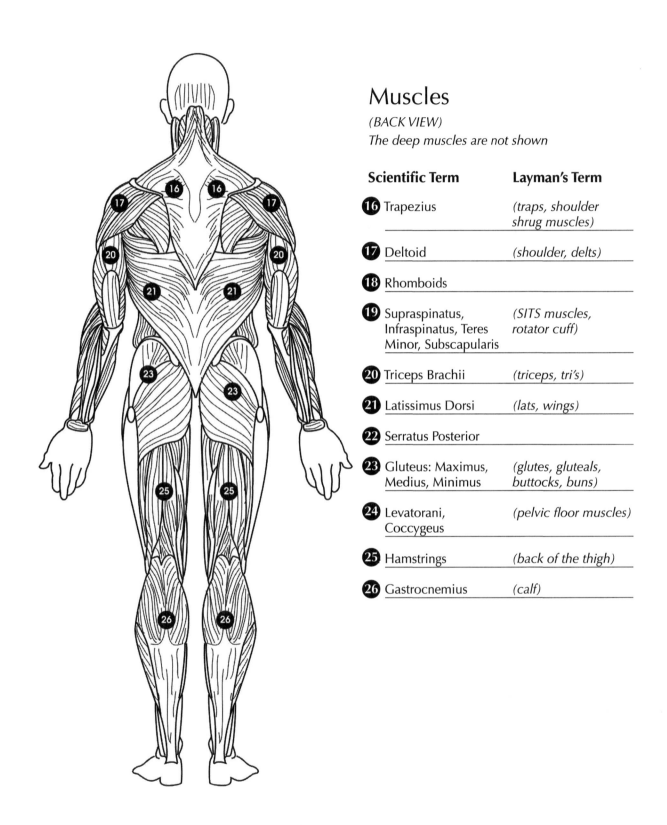

Muscles

(BACK VIEW)
The deep muscles are not shown

Scientific Term	Layman's Term
16 Trapezius	*(traps, shoulder shrug muscles)*
17 Deltoid	*(shoulder, delts)*
18 Rhomboids	
19 Supraspinatus, Infraspinatus, Teres Minor, Subscapularis	*(SITS muscles, rotator cuff)*
20 Triceps Brachii	*(triceps, tri's)*
21 Latissimus Dorsi	*(lats, wings)*
22 Serratus Posterior	
23 Gluteus: Maximus, Medius, Minimus	*(glutes, gluteals, buttocks, buns)*
24 Levatorani, Coccygeus	*(pelvic floor muscles)*
25 Hamstrings	*(back of the thigh)*
26 Gastrocnemius	*(calf)*

Skeleton

(FRONT VIEW)

Scientific Term	Layman's Term
1 Skull	*(head)*
2 Clavical	*(collar bone)*
3 Sternum	*(breast bone)*
4 Xiphoid Process	
5 Humerus	*(arm bone, upper arm)*
6 Elbow	*(funny bone)*
7 Ulna	*(forearm, lower arm)*
8 Radius	*(forearm, lower arm)*
9 Carpals, Metacarpals, Phalanges	*(hand, fingers)*
10 Ribcage, Thoracic Cage	*(ribs)*
11 Pelvic Girdle	*(pelvis, pelvic bone, hips)*
12 Ilium	
13 Anterior Superior Iliac Spine	*(hip bones, ASIS)*
14 Pubis Symphysis	*(pubic bone)*
15 Greater Trochanter	*(ball of femur)*
16 Femur	*(thigh bone, upper leg)*
17 Patella	*(knee cap)*
18 Tibia	*(leg bone, lower leg, shins)*
19 Fibula	*(leg bone, lower leg, shins)*
20 Tarsals, Metatarsals	*(foot, toes)*

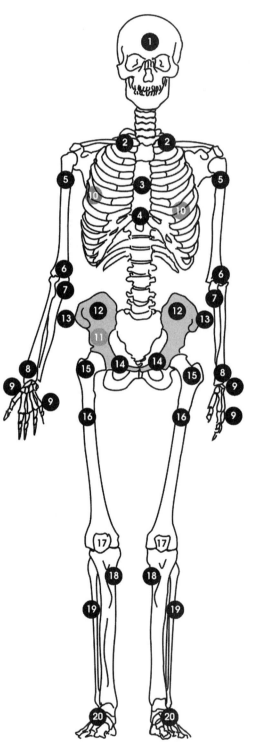

Skeleton

(BACK VIEW)

Scientific Term	**Layman's Term**
21 Scapula	*(shoulder blades)*
22 Vertebral Column	*(spine)*
23 (7) Cervical Vertebrae	*(neck)*
24 (12) Thoracic Vertebrae	*(middle of the back, behind the ribcage)*
25 (5) Lumbar Vertebrae	*(lower back)*
26 Iliac Crest	
27 Posterior Superior Iliac Spine	*(PSIS)*
28 Sacrum	
29 Coccyx, Coccygeal	*(tailbone)*
30 Ischium (Ischial Tuberosity)	*(sit-bones, sitz bones)*
31 Calcaneus	(heel)

Glossary

Abdominal Muscles: The elastic-like muscles layered across the midriff. These muscle fibers crisscross to form an anatomical girdle. They lie across each other at various angles. There are four groups: the rectus abdominis, external obliques, internal obliques, and transversus abdominis. These muscles attach to your ribcage and your pelvis. The muscles provide trunk stability and mobility. In Pilates they are referred to as your Powerhouse. The Foundation Exercise in Chapter Five assists you in contracting the deep postural abdominals toward your spine.

Abduction: The limbs move away from the midline of the body.

Adduction: The limbs move toward the midline of the body.

Alignment: Arrangement in a straight line.

Arabesque: A ballet term in which the leg is lifted and straightened backwards behind the body.

Attitude: A ballet term describing when the leg bends forward, sideways, or backwards.

Ballet Arms: The arms are extended but slightly curved, like hugging a big ball.

Beats: Beats are performed with the body in many positions. The legs come together with rhythmical accents. They cross at the ankle. Leg beats are a scissor-like motion guided by the contraction of your abdominal, buttock, and leg muscles.

Bound Flow: Controlled stops and starts of a sequence of movements. T'ai Chi is an example of bound flow movements—they are slow, smooth, and controlled.

Bridging, or Hinging: You are lying on your back to prepare for bridging. The soles of the feet are flat on the mat. The tailbone lifts first.

The hips rise. Roll successively through the spine, bone by bone. Finish at the level of your shoulder blades. Reverse, rolling back down one vertebra at a time.

Brush: The sole of the foot slides along the mat surface with dynamic force. The downward motion of your foot gives your leg the assistance to rise. Imagine brushing the foot deep into the mat systematically—heel, arch, ball, and toes—then the leg rises. This feeling of grounding helps an athlete or dancer push off into the air and land. It enhances balance.

Cat: A kneeling yoga posture on all fours. The trunk is curled in a C-shape. The spine is in flexion. The contraction of your abdominals supports the spine.

C-curve: The shape of the spine when the body is curled or in trunk flexion. This position is supported by the abdominals.

Center, or Centering: The human body has a physical center which includes the abdominals, back, hips, and buttocks muscles. The center is also referred to as the Powerhouse in Pilates. All motion ideally originates from the center. Centering means there is balance and control no matter what position the body is in, or how the limbs are moving. Pilates focuses on strengthening this area to support the spine and internal organs. The result is better posture.

Child Pose: This is a yoga posture. The body is in a low kneel. The trunk is folded over the legs. The head rests toward the floor. The arms are by your sides.

Cobra: A yoga posture lying on your stomach. Your hands are beneath the shoulders. Your upper body rises into spine extension (arch). Support this movement by contracting your abdominal muscles and the base of your Powerhouse—buttocks, pelvic floor, and upper thighs. The back of your neck stays long.

Core: Your core involves your trunk muscles: the abdominal, back, and buttock muscles. Establishing a strong core is the foundation of Pilates training. As these muscles get stronger your posture will improve. Core stabilizers are the smaller, deeper functional muscles that are closer to the bones. Their role is to improve coordination by stabilizing the skeletal system, and aligning the body. The larger structural muscles are the superficial muscles just beneath the skin. They provide power for moving the body through space.

Corset: The physical and mental act of the abdominals contracting to support the body. This helps you engage the Powerhouse. Visualize your ribcage area as a corset. The corset cinches together in front to help you expel air and support the spine.

Diaphragm: Muscle in your midriff that contracts to draw air into the lungs, and rises up to push air out of the lungs.

Dynamic Breathing: Pilates also refers to it as ribcage, lateral, or thoracic breathing. The aim is to keep the abdominal and spinal muscles engaged while the ribcage expands on inhalation. On the exhalation the ribcage contracts downward toward the waistline and involves the deep pelvic muscles.

Dynamic: The body's energetic output during the performance of movements.

Extend: Straightening.

Extension: A ballet term for stretching or lengthening the leg.

External Rotation: To turn a limb outwards or laterally away from the midline of the body.

Flexion: Bending.

Flow: Movements are performed like the flowing transitions of a dance. There are no jerky, uncontrolled movements.

Force: The dynamics of movement. The way one expends or controls energy during movements. The body's joint and muscular action controls the force. The quantity of energy affects the quality of the resulting movement.

Foundation Exercise: An exercise utilizing the muscular action of the abdominals in combination with the power of dynamic breathing to activate your center or Powerhouse. This exercise uses visualization to picture each layer of the abdominal muscles to build a strong foundation for all movements. The results are deep inward contractions of your abdominal muscles, and therefore strong, toned stomach muscles.

Free Flow: Movements with a continuous sequence of body action.

Gesture Leg or Arm: The leg or arm that does not support the body's weight. It is usually moving, but sometimes it is held in a position.

Girdle: The physical and mental act of the abdominals contracting to support the body to stand upright, move the limbs, and expel air. It helps activate the Powerhouse.

Grounding: A term used in sports, dance, and the martial arts. It refers to the power that emanates from a connection of the body into the ground. Grounding is evident when you watch a proficient tennis player. They know how to use their body and the court surface to make quick and efficient changes in direction, to get down, to bend their knees, to lunge for a ball, to reach, to pull up and away from the ground.

Horizontal: The human body moves in the horizontal direction side to side. These are like a basketball guard's lateral movements.

Internal Rotation: To turn a limb inwards or medially toward the midline of the body.

Kinetics: The scientific study of forces and energy on moving objects.

Lateral Breathing: Pilates term for an inhalation in which the ribcage inflates and expands side to side and into the back. The intercostal muscles in between the individual ribs stretch. As you exhale, bring the front ribs back together.

Lateral Flexion: A sideways bend.

Momentum: The force with which you exert movements. No exercise is uncontrolled. The momentum for each movement starts in your center or Powerhouse.

Navel To Spine: The physical and mental act of connecting your abdominals to your spine. This engages the muscles of the Powerhouse.

Neutral Pelvic Posture: The position in which the spine is in its natural state. Lie down on your back in order to find "neutral." Flatten your lower back to the floor and then slightly arch it away from the floor. Neutral is the comfortable place in between these two positions. This position provides safety for all movements.

Oppositional Lengthening: Moving the body in two different directions simultaneously to engage more muscle groups. Utilizing oppositional lengthening helps you to discover that your center abdominal area is not something you grab onto to hold a position. Instead, there is an ongoing interchange of motion from the abdominals to the limbs and back again. This helps you stretch and feel your body moving through space with confidence.

Parallel: In standing, the legs are aligned with the hip joints. The feet and the knees face forward.

Passé: A ballet term meaning to bring the gesture foot to the knee of the support leg.

Pelvic Floor: The bones and muscles located at the base of the pelvis. This is the area between the pubic bone and tailbone. It supports the internal organs. The base of the Powerhouse consists of this area along with the buttocks and upper thighs. Cough to feel the pelvic floor muscles.

Pilates Stance: The heels and legs are glued together. The feet are pointed yet relaxed. Turn out your legs slightly. External rotation occurs within the hip joint. Tighten your buttocks and wrap the backs of the thighs toward each other.

Powerhouse: The name Joseph Pilates gave to the abdominal area between the ribs and hips. These are the bands of muscles that encircle the torso. The Powerhouse includes a large group of muscles in our center—the abdomen, lower back, hips, and buttocks.

Prone: Lying face downward.

Sagittal: Movements forward and backward, like a fencer thrusting a sword.

Scoop: The act of pulling your navel into your spine by contracting the abdominal muscles. This creates a scooped-out appearance in the belly.

Shape: The design the body takes in space.

Shoulder Blades, Scapula: The pair of triangular bones lying on either side of the upper back. They are the principal bones of the shoulder girdle and articulate with the collarbone. The shoulder blades can glide up (elevation) and down (depression), in toward the spine (retraction), away from the spine (protraction), and can rotate upward and downward. Pull your shoulders slightly back. Then gently slide your shoulder blades downward. This makes more space between your ears and shoulders. It reduces neck and shoulder tension. Maintain this shoulder girdle organization as you exercise.

Shoulder Girdle Organization: The upper trunk muscles connect the arms to the body. This structure stabilizes the upper body so the arms can move with ease.

Sit-bones: These are the bones located at the base of the pelvis, which you sit on. You locate them by sitting and rocking side to side.

Space: The body's use of directions, pathways, and levels in space. For example, the directions: forward/backwards, the pathways: straight/curvy, and the levels: low/medium/high.

Spine Extension: The trunk arches.

Spine Flexion: The trunk curls.

Squeeze the Buttocks: This is the physical action of contracting the buttocks, back of the upper legs, inner thighs, and the pelvic floor muscles. Pilates refers to these areas as the base of your Powerhouse. These muscles can help you access your abdominals or Powerhouse.

Supine: Lying on the back.

Support Leg or Arm: This is the leg or arm that holds the body's weight or stabilizes the body. It can be moving or placed upon the mat.

Synovial Fluid: The body's natural version of oil for the joints. It protects the joints. This fluid is activated through exercise.

Three-Dimensional Breathing: The mental and physical act of exercising your breathing muscles—the diaphragm, chest, and ribs. The practice of this exercise increases lung capacity. It replaces the habit of shallow chest breathing with deep diaphragmatic breathing. Visualization provides the intention for stretching the inner volumes within the body—in the vertical, horizontal, and sagittal directions. This breathing pattern reinforces the use of dynamic breathing for more core control.

Time: Movements have a rate of speed. Intervals or pulse beats can be measured as in music. Time can be slow, moderate, or fast. Also, your attitude toward timing can be dictated by the nature of the movement itself, breathing rhythms, or the ebb and flow of energy.

Vertebra (plural, Vertebrae): Bony segments that make up the spinal column.

Visual Imagery: The use of a mental picture to accomplish physical tasks. This is an essential element of dance, sports, Pilates, and stress management. It helps the mind more effectively control the body. Visual imagery trains the brain to create new neurological pathways. It enhances muscular coordination. This is referred to as muscle memory. The result is improved efficiency of motion, motor control, posture, and the knowledge of where your body is in space. Dancers, athletes, and Pilates participants use visualization to accentuate the mind-body connection. It leads to success in attaining mastery over new physical skills. It enhances artistic expression.

Vertical: Up and down movements, like a tennis player's serve.

Z-sit: Sit with the legs bent. This is a sitting position in which both of the legs are swept to one side of the body. The front foot is against the back knee.

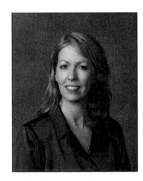

Larkin Barnett has spent thirty years teaching, lecturing, choreographing, and performing for several organizations including Harvard University, Radcliffe College, Longy School of Music, the Laban Bartenieff Institute, the University of Lappeenranta, Mills College, Canyon Ranch Spa, and the Johnson and Johnson Corporation. She was a professor of dance at Virginia Commonwealth University. Ms. Barnett was personally selected by Harvard University to direct and choreograph a commissioned project sponsored through the Harvard Fund For The Arts.

Larkin has given lectures and workshops in the dance and Pilates-based Life Extension System at Canyon Ranch Spa, where she was a fitness trainer, and had a private movement therapy practice.

Larkin is the Director of Pilates for the Ray Floyd Old Palm Golf Club and live-in community. She also teaches in the Health Sciences Department at Florida Atlantic University. Larkin holds several Pilates certifications from different governing organizations, including International Polestar Education. She also has two certifications in Pilates for golf. Ms. Barnett's credentials include a B.A. in Dance and Drama from Sweet Briar College, and an M.A. in Dance from Mills College.